Communicating in Dental Practice:
Stress-Free Dentistry and Improved Patient Care

Communicating in Dental Practice: Stress-Free Dentistry and Improved Patient Care

By
Ruth Freeman
Gerry Humphris

Editor-in-Chief: Nairn H F Wilson
Editor Operative Dentistry: Paul A Brunton

Quintessence Publishing Co. Ltd.
London, Berlin, Chicago, Paris, Milan, Barcelona, Istanbul,
São Paulo, Tokyo, New Delhi, Moscow, Prague, Warsaw

British Library Cataloguing-in Publication Data

Freeman, Ruth, Dr
 Communicating in dental practice: stress-free dentistry and improved patient care.
 - (Quintessentials of dental practice; 30)
 1. Communication in dentistry 2. Dental personnel and patient
 I. Title II. Humphris, Gerry III. Wilson, Nairn H. F. IV. Brunton, Paul A.
 617.6

ISBN 1850970998

Illustrators: Laura Andrew & Abi Le Santo

ISBN 1-85097-099-8

Foreword

Effective communicating is fundamental to success in clinical practice. Indeed, many tensions between patients and members of the dental team, in particular complaints, stem from failures in communications.

There is a great deal more to communicating in healthcare provision than simply applying interpersonal skills and techniques developed in everyday life. This important volume in the multifaceted *Quintessentials* series provides great insight into key communication skills and techniques of special relevance to the dental team. Following consideration of basic and advanced communication skills, with reference to special dental situations, the authors – international leaders in the field – focus in on major communication challenges in clinical practice, such as communicating effectively with anxious, "difficult" and dissatisfied patients, communicating and integrating preventive and oral health messages and education in primary dental care, and ways in which patient care can be improved without adding to the stress of frontline clinical practice.

This excellent addition to the unique *Quintessential* series is both a springboard and stimulus to communicating more effectively – a means to less stress, fewer complaints, improved clinical outcomes and patients who better understand their problems and appreciate their oral healthcare. It is not always what you do, but how you communicate it! The evening or two it will take to read this carefully crafted book will be time well spent.

Nairn Wilson
Editor-in-Chief

Acknowledgements

We would like to thank Catherine Coyle for providing the example of communicating with a boy with Asperger's syndrome.

Contents

Chapter 1
Introduction

Dentistry can be a rewarding and satisfying profession. Dental health professionals must have a variety of skills to hand. These include not only clinical and technical skills but also those associated with patient management, managerial and financial acumen. This is reflected in their financial remuneration, which is often above average for staff employed within health-related disciplines. The principals of practices and, to a lesser extent, associates, have the ability to work at a pace they can ultimately decide upon. In reality this may seem something of a fantasy, as the demands on the modern practitioner appear less amenable to individual control. However, on closer inspection there are demands other than the financial and management constraints of running a busy practice that can cause difficulties. Some of these problems relate to patient and staff interaction and include the following:

- difficult and demanding patients
- encouraging patients to adhere to oral health recommendations
- managing pain
- the dentally anxious patient
- patients with unexplained symptoms
- informing patients about oral health, self-care and specialist treatments.

The aim of this book is to signpost principles and actions that will enhance the process of communication with patients and mitigate many of the difficulties listed above. The book will provide a framework within a dental context to assist with understanding the complex set of factors that make up dental practice in the 21st century. The authors have distilled the current literature into an authoritative account, with a small number of key references listed at the end of each chapter, including selected further reading.

What Makes this Book Different?

This volume translates recognised psychological and sociological principles into everyday clinical practice. The emphasis will be on application to the day-to-day working of the dental health professional. Hence, a major theme throughout the book will be communication between the dentist and the patient. Enhancement of an appropriate working relationship is a central focus. Less space will be devoted to systems of care outside the practice (for example, health organisations, mass media interventions and oral health surveys).

Self-care is a neglected subject in the health professions. The professional and philosophical underpinnings of primary dental care have tended to diminish the need to maintain good physical and psychological health of its practitioners while concentrating efforts on improving patient care. The authors would prefer to redress the balance and advocate the need of practitioners to ensure that they care for themselves enough to:

• maintain high standards of care for patients
• develop new techniques of prevention and treatment as they come on stream
• achieve longer-term personal goals and therefore become more resilient to the vagaries of occupational stress and burnout
• be able to recognise physical and emotional problems associated with work and outside the workplace.

Occupational stress is an easily recognised phenomenon in modern dental practice. However, the term has a tendency to be overused, or simply raised without further discussion of some of the underlying reasons for its experience for many working in dental practice. Alternatively, causative agents that can be championed conveniently (such as the remuneration system) exclude the individual practitioners and the means at their disposal to at least attempt to minimise some of these pressures. The reader is invited to accept the possibility that many of the day-to-day hassles that feature in practitioners' work can be analysed and interpreted from the interaction that occurs between patient and practitioner.

Section 1: Communication

This section comprises three chapters (Chapters 2-4). Chapter 2 deals with different aspects of communication. Practitioners may be familiar with many of the fundamental building blocks of communication skills utilised in dentist-patient interactions. These basic skills are cornerstones that lend themselves to repeated attention and practice in the workplace. Even the simple application of a well-placed or considered greeting can pay dividends to the overall satisfaction and outcome from the patient's perspective. Hence, these skills are described and illustrated from the dental practice perspective.

Chapter 3 expands the communication theme by identifying important areas of clinical practice that command excellent use of advanced communication

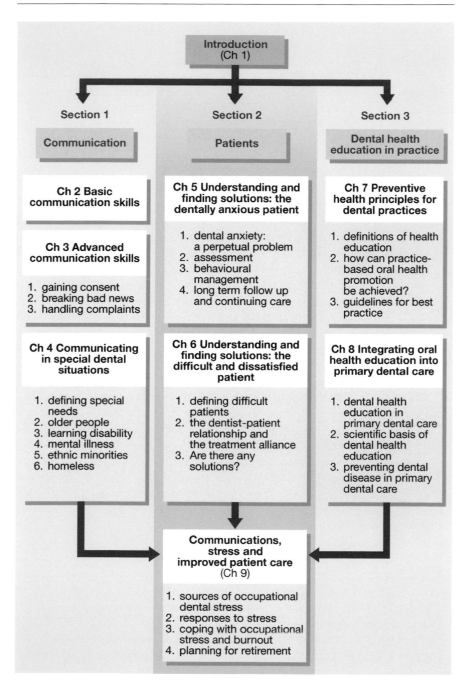

skills. Negotiating with patients various options available for treatment entails a complex blend of skills to ensure cooperation and adherence to the eventual agreed plan.

Obtaining consent for treatment requires sensitive handling to ensure that patients are fully conversant with the implications of their decision to embark on a treatment, including possibilities of success or failure and any side-effects. Included in these discussions, in all probability, will be estimates of costs of care and requests for payment (under fee for item, insurance payment or private contract schemes). An additional area of communication often confronted by clinicians is the breaking of bad news to patients. This may take the form of simply announcing to a patient that a tooth requires extraction. The meaning associated with the tooth loss can be assessed with a well-chosen open-ended question. Alternatively, providing unwelcome news to patients may take the form of a potentially frightening opinion, such as a suspicious lesion under the tongue, indicative of an oral squamous cell carcinoma. Admittedly, this is a very infrequent circumstance, but one that dentists have stated as being one of the most stressful incidents in their working lives. It is assumed that practitioners who think about these scenarios and hopefully practise their skills in continuing professional development training events will improve their competency and also confidence.

Patient expectations are known to be increasing in the health care field. Without clear explanations of procedures and realistic estimates of outcome and costs the clinician will be prone to complaint. Even the most diligent and competent clinician will be exposed to the risk of treatment unexpectedly failing. Human error is, unfortunately, a feature of health service provision and requires sensitive handling and management. Over 90% of litigation in the health service has been attributed to poor communication skills. Some key points can be offered to the practitioner to prevent a complaint escalating into formal action (considered by the majority of dentists to be the most extreme stressor).

Chapter 4, the last of this first section of the book, extends the discussion of communication skills applied in certain situations to focusing on particular groups of patients. It is acknowledged that the identification of a patient group by attaching a label has negative connotations. For example, the 'elderly', a term sometimes applied to those over the age of 60, can introduce punitive stereotyping and discrimination. To make some generalisations for a particular group can, however, be illuminating if the practitioner is aware that the group profile will vary according to the individual presentation of the patient and that the requirements of the individual should remain paramount. The communication skills associated with the following groups will be described: older people, people with physical and learning difficulties.

Section 2: Patients

The second section, consisting of two chapters, focuses on the patient. A whole chapter (Chapter 5) is devoted to the anxious patient, who has been acknowledged as one of the most frequent and demanding types of patient the practitioner will meet. Much has been written about the assessment and management of the dentally anxious patient. The approach adopted in this chapter will summarise the recognised methods of identifying the anxious and phobic patient and suggested ways of encouraging successful treatment and continued access to the dental practice for long-term oral health care.

The second chapter (Chapter 6) of this patient section introduces the management of patients with difficulties that are not necessarily dental in origin but are expressed as oral symptoms or problems. Without a considered assessment and understanding of the complexities of the presenting symptoms and complaints, the practitioner may be drawn into unnecessary treatment or referral for further investigations. Attention to detailed history taking and formation of the treatment alliance (working relationship) are important features in providing appropriate care from the dental practice setting.

Section 3: Dental Health Education in Practice

The last section, consisting of two chapters, presents key material for practitioners to conduct, essentially, one-to-one dental health education with their patients. This work rests on the ability of the practitioner to communicate effectively (a central theme of this book) and to be aware of the substantial advances and benefits to patients available from adoption of these approaches. Chapter 7 presents a number of the extant models that have influenced dental health education over the years. They have been drawn from various areas and have had proven value in improving patient knowledge, beliefs and behaviour in relation to dental health behaviours such as toothbrushing, diet control and dental attendance.

Chapter 8 continues with a series of examples where these models have been applied in one form or another. The evidence base for many of these preventive interventions is commented upon. Benefits can be demonstrated with one-to-one approaches in dental health education. All members of a practice should work to the same preventive protocol to have a synergistic effect. Furthermore, developing a preventive philosophy for the practice will provide additional outcomes for the general dental practitioner (for example, reduced stress) and the patient (for example, quality of life).

Chapter 9 concludes the book by returning to the major theme of improving patient care through the maintenance of self-care and practice of excellent communication skills. In reality, problems occur both personally and in the workplace. Practitioners are given ways of assessing themselves to indicate whether a problem may exist (for example, burnout or excessive drinking). It is the expected outcome of this book for the reader to appreciate and adopt communication skills and self-care actions to improve service delivery to patients visiting the dental practice based in primary care.

Chapter 2
Basic Communication Skills

Aim

To present the fundamental building blocks and processes of communication between dental personnel and patients.

Outcome

After reading this chapter the reader will understand the components of communication skills and have guidance on when to use each skill appropriately.

The Importance of Clinical Communication Skills

A fundamental skill for the practising dentist is to be able to communicate well with patients and members of the dental team. For many health professionals there is good agreement that being able to communicate is central to assessing patient needs, providing information and gaining compliance. With the provision of ever more complex treatments and a drive towards comprehensive dental care, these skills may become 'automatic', and bad habits develop as attention is focused on technical or administrative areas. Good communication skills prevent complaints (see Chapter 3), increase acceptance of treatment decisions and adherence to recommendations. Communication is key to successful dentist-patient interaction and can contribute to a thriving dental practice. It consists of:
• introducing oneself to patients and staff
• appreciating the importance of non-verbal communication
• use of language appropriate to persons and situations
• use of open and closed questions
• proximity and the special case of dental practice
• empathic responding
• explaining and advising.

Communication skills divide naturally into two major categories divided by the use of words as opposed to actions without words. These two categories and constituent behaviours are summarised in Table 2-1.

Table 2-1 **The two major areas of communication skills**

Verbal	Non-verbal
Explaining	Body language
Questioning	Eye contact
Listening	Proximity and personal space
Clarifying	Level and posture
Repeating	Non-verbal cues
Goal setting	Tone, volume, rate of speech

By careful questioning and effective listening the dentist can uncover difficulties patients have experienced and establish how they feel in the dental setting. By watching and observing the patient's non-verbal behaviours (NVBs), the dentist can assess:
• the patient's emotional state
• how consistent the patient's NVBs match the content of what the patient says.

Therefore the communication skills a dentist utilises should enable him/her to satisfy the following clinical goals:
• create the right atmosphere to establish rapport
• encourage patients to volunteer information and to feel involved in their own care
• identify and negotiate dental health goals with the patient
• use a style and language that is appropriate to each particular patient at each stage of the interaction
• recognise when an interview is going wrong and make appropriate adjustments
• seek the patient's compliance with treatment plans and health goals.

Six key elements of communication have been identified:
1. understanding non-verbal communication
2. listening

3. engaging people to talk
4. asking questions and obtaining feedback
5. acknowledging other people's feelings
6. giving feedback.

The skills involved in questioning, explaining and listening are fundamental to interviewing techniques. Communication is usually thought of as a two-way process in which the dentist initially appears to be passive, listening, and the patient active, talking. This is initially an unfamiliar situation for both dentist and patient, since the dentist is often active and the patient passive – an apparent reversal of roles. Further difficulties arise as the patient may feel that the dentist is being critical or judgmental while the dentist may feel that s/he is being supportive and tactful in approach.

Other problems arise in communication as a result of time in consultation and the confines of the dental surgery. Both of these can cause distortion of the communication process, which can be further exacerbated by:-
- the equipment in the surgery presenting a clinical and impersonal environment
- patients' reluctance to express their feelings, thoughts and anxieties (the patient may feel that this area is not the domain of the dental consultation process)
- the dentist adopting a rigid question–and–answer format that becomes overly formulaic.

The dentist must listen actively, processing what the patient is saying, meaning and feeling. In addition, he or she must make educated guesses of what the patient may be avoiding to say and encourage him or her to feel able to reveal a particular concern or special request. The dentist must keenly use and perfect these skills of questioning, explaining and listening to the patient.

Questioning

Questions are used to try to find out more about patients' needs, wants, feelings and so on. Different types or categories of question exist and lie along a continuum. Each of these question categories is used for different purposes.

Open Questions
An open question is designed to enable the patient to answer in a variety of ways. 'How are you today?' or 'How do you feel about dental treatment?'

are good examples. They are typically used at the beginning of the consultation and facilitate information gathering.

Open questions allow the patient:
- to talk. The patient is in control and can bring as much or as little information s/he feels is necessary, or wishes to impart, to the interview
- to set the agenda
- to vent anxieties and concerns.

Focused Questions
This type of questioning restricts the content of the patient's reply. Focused questions:
- guide the interview/conversation
- help patients to tell the health professional more about a topic they have difficulty in speaking about
- are used to obtain difficult or sensitive information. A typical wording [with explanatory note in square brackets] would be: 'I appreciate that it is hard to tell me [an open intention] about subject X [guidance or direction] but you must try [support].'

Examples:
- 'Tell me more about the pain. What is it like?'
- 'Why do you think you are so frightened about having an injection?'

Closed Questions
They are the most frequently used questions in a history-taking interview to focus on specific topics.

Closed questions:
- help to clarify important points brought to the interview/conversation by the patient
- are sometimes described as yes/no questions. Usually there is only a yes or no answer
- are usually used late in the interview to clarify. If used too early in the conversation the patient will be unable to volunteer information and will just answer your questions, in order to be helpful.

Examples:
- 'Is it the tooth at the back that has been keeping you awake at night?'
- 'Have you ever had growing pains? Sometimes people call this chorea or rheumatic fever.'

General Guidelines for Questioning

1. Take time to think before you speak.
2. Move between open, focused, and closed questions during the conversation.
3. Avoid jargon. However, if used it is important to be sure that the patient understands you.
4. Ask one question at a time.
5. Leading questions are to be avoided. Patients can feel so intimidated that even if they do not understand what you are saying they will say 'yes'.

Explaining

Explaining or giving advice to patients is a vital part of the work of the health professional. It is used to:
• negotiate health goals
• instruct self-care procedures at home
• outline new treatment procedure prior to agreeing to consent.

Some frameworks have been devised that include good practice and have been summarised as mnemonics - for example, SMARTIS or ARMPITS, presented later (see Chapter 7). A set of 10 guidelines to encourage better explaining and advice giving are presented in Table 2-2. Perhaps the most important thing about explaining is clarity - that is, for the practitioner to be quite clear about the objectives. Some questions you might ask yourself before you talk to a patient are:
• What changes do you want the patient to make?
• What do you want the patient to know, feel, be able to do?

Listening

The third, and probably the most important of communication skills, is active listening. General medical practitioners have been shown to allow their patients only 20 seconds on average to reveal the reason for their visit before interjecting. Hence, listening requires at the very least that the dentist gives patients a reasonable time to convey their views or set of symptoms. Listening is not, however, simply allowing space for the patient to speak and hearing the words being spoken. It also involves a concerted effort:
• to listen to the way the words are said
• to be conscious of the feelings underlying the words spoken

11

Table 2-2 **General guidelines for explaining and giving advice**

Top 10 'tips' for explaining information to patients

1. Be realistic in the objectives you set - give only three or four key points.

2. Advice and instructions should be given early in the session –most important information should be given first.

3. Emphasise those items that are the most important - repeat key points.

4. Use short words and sentences.

5. Avoid jargon - ensure that technical words are understood.

6. Information is best given in a structured way; that is, 'chunk' the message into a number of discrete points.

7. Use visual aids [health education posters, leaflets or mouth/tooth models] where possible, to support what you are saying.

8. Check during explanation that patient comprehends your message and allow them to ask for clarification.

9. Put patient at ease by assessing if they are dentally anxious or have any worries.

10. Be friendly - not officious – sufficient to establish rapport.

- to recognise hidden feelings
- to be aware of what is left unsaid.

Often the main task of the listener is to help the person to express himself or herself. Again specific skills are involved in this. These are:
- encouraging the patient to talk
- giving attention to what is being said - being interested in the patient
- reflecting feelings - for instance, 'you seem pleased' or 'upset'

- paraphrasing – the patient's words to clarify what s/he has been telling you
- summing up – a brief summing-up of the main content and feelings the patient has alluded to during the interview.

Listening also involves being aware of non-verbal communications. This is important, since 65% of all social interactions are made up of non-verbal communications. Non-verbal cues are more readily believed than verbal statements of intent – 'actions speak louder than words'.

Non-verbal behaviour of the clinician can affect clients' ability to cope with dental experiences. Patients can also demonstrate their feelings to the dental team through this channel of communication. Some of the non-verbal aspects of communication that dental health professionals need to be aware of are:

Level/Position
Refers to differences in height between people, whether people are sitting, standing or lying. The patient who is lying in the dental chair can feel uncomfortable, vulnerable and at a disadvantage to the dental practitioner who may be standing. In practice, when assessing patients' opinions about their oral health or treatment, the patient should be seated upright with the dentist sitting (on the wheel-mounted stool) alongside.

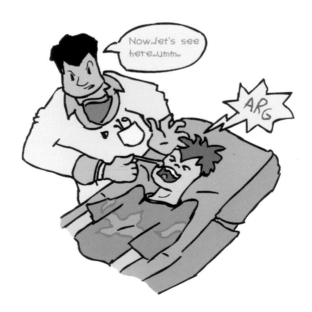

Proximity

Refers to how close people are to one another. In certain social situations the invasion of a person's personal space is disconcerting and unacceptable; at other times it is acceptable and welcomed. In dentistry the patient allows the dentist permission to invade his/her social space for the delivery of treatment. This invasion of space is given implicitly by the patient. It relies on a trusting relationship being established and maintained.

Posture

Refers to how people stand, sit, lie or 'hold themselves'. Posture can indicate whether the patient is relaxed, uneasy or anxious. For instance, a young girl lying in the dental chair with her knees drawn up to her chest signals to the dentist how anxious she feels.

Eye Contact

This is an important first step in establishing rapport with a patient. This can convey to patients that the dental health professional is interested, willing to understand their needs and feels empathy for them. Patients who avoid making eye contact with the dentist are often frightened of dental treatment, the dentist's response to their behaviour or are anxious about what they have to say.

Non-Verbal Reinforcers of Speech

These include tone, pitch, speed of talking and can indicate feelings including anger, fear and doubt. Another indicator of anxiety is referred to as 'ahs', 'ers' and 'uhms'. These filled pauses indicate that the patient is trying to find words to convey his/her feelings or doubts to the dentist.

Conclusions

Communication has been referred to as the heart of the consultation between patient and dentist. It is often relegated to 'the wings' rather than being 'centre stage' in the consultation, simply through neglect, apathy and the development of bad habits in the hope of cutting corners and saving time. The 'patient-centred' care movement has been successful in reversing this trend by developing an evidence base for health care professionals to adopt good practice. Central to this process has been the core construct of listening to patients and respecting their account of events, feelings and requirements. Evidence from the broader clinical communication literature has shown that patient-centred care need not necessarily lengthen appointment times. Paradoxically, over a series of appointments advantages accrue, including greater patient satisfaction, increased adherence to recommendations, fewer practice complaints and no overall increase in contact time. The dentist is encouraged to adopt these basic principles. Chapter 3 concentrates on more specific communication skills, focusing on ethically complex clinical scenarios.

Further Reading

Silverman J, Kurtz S, Draper J. Skills for Communicating with Patients. Abingdon: Radcliffe Medical Press, 1998.

Chapter 3
Advanced Communication Skills

Aim

To present guidelines for some common episodes within dental consultations that require advanced communication skills.

Outcome

By the end of this chapter the reader will be able to relate to an inclusive method of obtaining consent from patients, breaking bad news and dealing with complaints and solving problems. Moreover, recommendations on how to give bad news to patients will be outlined.

Obtaining Consent

To embark on treatment the dentist requires consent from the patient to proceed. Traditionally this process has depended on the dentist making a diagnosis of the patient's disease and then constructing a treatment plan. At this stage the patient would be told of the condition and proposed treatment and, if the patient voiced no objections, the work would begin. The General Dental Council has placed increasing emphasis on consent, and a more interactive approach is advocated. This deliberately involves the patient in the decision-making process. Dentists have mixed views about obtaining consent. Estimates of the amount of time spent gaining consent have shown that general dental practitioners (GDPs) spend seven minutes explaining and obtaining consent, whereas salaried and private dentists spend on average 11 minutes (King et al, 2000). Over 80% of dentists in a recent survey stated that they explained the problem, but less than half explained risks of treatment or checked patient understanding. Furthermore, less than a quarter actually obtained written consent. From the patient perspective it was found that a large majority felt they had received enough information about their dental problem (95%) and that the dentist had explained things well (78%). Six out of 10 patients stated that they had not been told about alternative treatments, and 42% were uncertain about when the treatment would be completed.

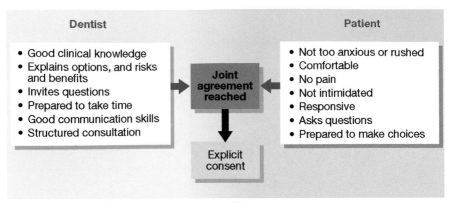

Fig 3-1 Factors making consent more explicit.

There are advantages from following a comprehensive consent procedure (see Fig 3-1).

The communication skills employed when obtaining consent are numerous and have to be coordinated. Ensure that the procedure occurs when you and the patient are seated together, preferably at the same level so that eye contact can be made with little effort. Have pencil and paper to hand to assist with explanations of dental problems and possible treatments and to summarise risks, estimates and costs. Offer leaflets as back-up material to aid explanation.

It is easy in this process to rush on ahead, in particular with time scheduling in mind. Time spent on the consenting procedure will save time in subsequent sessions. Hence at each stage check with the patient that s/he is clear about what you have said. Patients will perceive this process as very supportive - in particular if all members of the dental team adopt this 'checking' approach. Of course, if patients are asked for their comments or questions then they must be given space in the process to respond. There is a temptation to ask the patient questions and to launch forward before s/he can muster their thoughts and reply.

The suggested model, outlined above (Table 3-1), proposed by King et al (2000) identifies procedures for dentists to obtain consent from patients who have little difficulty in comprehension. Other patients - for example, those with learning difficulties, from other cultures, or from vulnerable groups (young or old people) - may demand special consideration. The involve-

Table 3-1 **Stages in the process of obtaining informed consent**

Interactive model	Consent in practice
Making introductions	Greeting patient and introducing oneself
Explaining the dental problem	Identifying problem
	Explaining problem in jargon-free language
Outlining various treatment options	Identifying treatments from examination and dental knowledge
	Explaining options simply
	Check if further explanation is needed
Discussing risks and benefits	Presenting benefits
	Presenting risks
	Check if need further explanation
Estimating time and costs	Discussing the issues of time and costs
Inviting questions	Ask for any questions
Reaching mutual understanding	Check if fully understands options and the reasons for choosing selected treatment
Confirming choices and agreement	Draw process to a close and obtain verbal agreement
Indicating consent (written)	Acquire signed consent and place this in patient's notes

ment of advocates, translators, carer and parents/relatives requires additional skills from the dental health professional (see Chapter 4). These include the careful listening to all the parties present when new information is explained. Difficulties can occur when the practitioner needs to make a decision on the behalf of another adult. In UK law the clinician has the right to decide for the patient the various treatments required. Although it would be prudent for the practitioner to invite opinion from the carer, the responsibility resides with the dentist to make the best treatment choice on behalf of the patient who is unable to select for him or herself. Every effort should be made to involve and encourage the patient and carer. Organisational assistance for this process can include:

- seating arrangements for carers as well as patients
- reduced periods of time in the waiting room
- ensure follow-up appointments are made routinely
- have a system for efficient waiting-list management.

Breaking Bad News: General Principles

- One person only should be responsible for breaking bad news.
- The person who breaks the bad news should be the lead clinician who is responsible for the patient's care.
- The patient has a legal and moral right to accurate, reliable information.
- The dentist's primary responsibility is to the individual patient (relatives or significant others are secondary). If necessary, use a professional interpreter for cultural or linguistic assistance.
- Give the patient accurate and reliable information so that s/he understands any implications.
- Always ask patients how much information they want about their prognosis.
- Information giving should be staged over more than one consultation rather than giving all the information at one time. It is difficult for patients to take in a lot of important information on a single occasion.
- Dentists should tell patients about bad news as early as possible in the diagnostic process rather than waiting to the end of the various test procedures.
- Make every attempt to tell the patient in person. Only in exceptional cases inform patients of bad news over the telephone.
- The dentist should ensure that the patient has support (relatives, close friend and so on) at the time of giving bad news.
- Provide sufficient time for the bad-news consultation.
- Tell the patient in private, in comfortable surroundings if at all possible,

and make arrangements not to be disturbed (by telephone or mobiles/ bleepers).

• Involve others by inviting the patient to nominate a family member to be present. Also ensure that another member of staff is present to listen and act as a support for the patient if you are not available at some future point. Ask the patient if this is acceptable.

General Principles for Handling Complaints and Solving Problems

• When a patient comes to you with a complaint or disagreement:
  - Discuss the problem as soon as possible. If time is not available then organise a mutually suitable appointment.
  - Adopt a polite and helpful manner; try not to react defensively, hurt- fully or angrily.
  - Hear the patient out. Listen carefully to the patient's words and espe- cially to the feelings expressed.

Steps taken for	Patient	Dentist
handling complaints & solving problems	focus	focus
Step 1	Let the patient state the problem	
Step 2		Listen carefully to the patient's concerns
Step 3		Apologise for distress caused Check your understanding of the problem by summarising
Step 4		Share your thoughts and feelings about the problem
Step 5	Brainstorm some solutions	
Step 6	Try to reach an agreement and be as specific as possible	

Fig 3-2 Handling complaints and solving problems.

21

- Remember, as your patient s/he has a right to complain. Complaints may help to improve the quality of your practice.

- Once the patient has finished speaking:
  - Apologise for the distress caused.
  - Summarise what s/he has said so that you have clarified and understood the problem.
  - Share your thoughts and feelings on the matter so that the patient can understand your point of view.
  - Discuss several proposals to remedy the problem. Try to be as specific as possible about what you can do to solve the problem.

- If a solution cannot be found:
  - It may be that you and the patient are mismatched.
  - Refer the patient to another dentist in the practice.
  - Remember to keep the complaints confidential.

- Maintain a detailed record of complaints, including dated accounts of discussions and outcomes.

Conclusions

The aim of this chapter was to provide practical guidelines to assist dentists in developing their communication skills. Three specific areas were examined - gaining consent, breaking bad news and handling complaints and problem-solving. It was suggested that these areas required advanced communication skills, and hence specific guidelines were provided. Communicating effectively with patients in difficult clinical encounters will lower fears of litigation and reduce occupational stress.

Further Reading

Further information on gaining consent and handling complaints can be found through membership of:
- Dental Protection – www.dentalprotection.org
- The DDU – www.the-DDU.com/dentist

King J, Doyal L, Hillier S. Consent in Dental Care. London: King's Fund Publishing, 2000.

Chapter 4
Communicating in Special Dental Situations

Aim

The aim of this chapter is to provide the reader with an understanding of how communication skills may be modified to match the requirements of patients with special dental needs. The communication skills described in Chapters 2 and 3 are the basis for this chapter. Practical suggestions will be described and how alterations of the basic concepts of communication can assist the dentist in the care of patients with special dental needs.

Outcome

At the end of this chapter the dentist should know the meaning of the terms impairment, disability and handicap, special needs and social exclusion. The dentist should have an awareness of the need to provide accessible information in both verbal and written form for patients with communication difficulties. The need for the use of interpreters for those with hearing impairment and/or children and adults with a learning disability is examined, together with the acknowledgement that the inclusion of a third person alters the dynamics of communicating with the patient. Mention is made of the communication programmes 'Writing with Symbols', Wigit© and Makaton©, and their usefulness when interacting with people with communication difficulties in the dental surgery.

Defining Special Needs

The term 'special needs' is difficult to define, as it has become associated with various different meanings. In 1980 the World Health Organization attempted to define special needs in terms of the terms impairment, disability and handicap:

- Impairment was defined as a loss or abnormality of bodily function and/or structure.
- Disability was defined as any restriction or lack of ability to execute an action considered to be within the normal range of human activity.
- Handicap was defined as a disadvantage as a result of the impairment or disability, which limited or prevented the individual experiencing and

Table 4-1 **Defining special needs**

Special needs as defined by the World Health Organization	Special needs as defined by the medical model	Special needs as defined by social exclusion
Impairment: a loss or abnormality of bodily function and or structure.	The individual has or is: Physical disability	Groups of people socially excluded by society:
	Learning difficulties	Disabled
Disability: any restriction or lack of ability to execute an action within the normal range of human activity.	Mental illness	Older people
	Medically compromised	Long-term sick
	Infectious diseases (for example, HIV)	Housebound
Handicap: a disadvantage as a result of the impairment or disability		Unemployed people
	Malignant diseases	Homeless people
	Dependent and/or terminally ill	Ethnic minorities

fulfilling all aspects of their lives as considered to be normal for that individual.

A result of the WHO definitions was to group all people with special needs together in accordance with the medical diagnosis of their impairment, disability, or handicap (Table 4-1). Furthermore, as these definitions relied heavily on the medical model they promoted the tendency to perceive special needs patients as 'ill'. An alternative definition existed, however. If disability was perceived within a social framework, special needs could be understood as a label society had provided for those who were impaired. Thinking in this way allowed the realisation that the label 'special need' belonged not with the disabled person but with society. It was society that branded individuals as having a special need and consequently excluded them from society, all types of services, social production and goods, resulting in economic exclusion.

Therefore people who are socially excluded may or may not be disabled but they may be unemployed, impoverished, homeless and may misuse alcohol and drugs. Social exclusion is a major factor in the increased prevalence of ill health found in these individuals. Therefore, while treating people with special needs may require a medical classification with regard to infection control or antibiotic cover, in order to reduce barriers and improve access to dental services dentists should perceive special needs within the parameters of social exclusion and societal demands. Thinking in this way improves access to care and communication for people with special dental needs.

The acknowledgement of the requirement for specialist training for dentists caring for patients with special dental needs has been recognised by the Royal College of Surgeons of England. The proposed new speciality of 'special care dentistry' has allowed the role of communication, behavioural sciences and health promotion to be seen as central in the oral health care of these patients. Information about the Diploma in Special Care Dentistry may be found at http://www.rcseng.ac.uk/dental/fds/examinations/pdf/regs_dscd.pdf

Are Patients with Special Dental Needs Treated in General Practice?

Evidence from work with general dental practitioners suggests that a variety of patients with special dental needs are treated in general dental practice. The majority of patients with hearing or sight impairment are readily accepted, as are older people and those with physical and learning disability. If the disability is regarded as too severe or the older person is too cognitively compromised the patient is referred to salaried primary dental or secondary dental services. The situation with regard to HIV-seropositive patients was different. One general practitioner stated: 'A patient of mine has just been diagnosed with HIV and asked if I would still treat him. There is no question about it – of course I will. I'm not taking on any new patients at the moment – and so I won't be taking on anyone, so it's not an issue of whether they are HIV-positive or not.'

The role of decision-making in general practice is discussed in Chapter 6 and how decisions may be made with regard to treatment and management. For the purposes of this chapter the assumption is made that the choice has been made to include the individual as a practice patient and necessitates a delivery of appropriate and effective communication skills.

Communicating with Older People

Life expectancy of people in the developed countries is increasing. This means that the proportion of older adults within communities is greater. The likelihood that these people will require continued dental care well into their eighth decade is now recognised. Improved oral health of people in their sixth decade has been shown to have an impact on service provision, since they expect high-quality dental care. Referred to as the 'young old', patients aged 65 to 74 will have experienced restorative dental care and expect more high-tech solutions than partial dentures for the replacement of missing teeth. The myth that older people will naturally loose teeth is being dispelled. Greater efforts are being made by patients themselves and their dentists to retain their natural dentition (rather than resort to partial or full dentures).

Dental practitioners and their staff will need to be encouraged and trained to prevent and counter-act long standing attitudes that may be prejudicial to the provision of holistic care for older people. Unfortunately, without awareness among some members of the dental team of negative behaviours towards older people (over the age of 64 years) it will be difficult to maintain a sensitive and competent caring regime for this group. Regrettably, it is common, for healthcare providers to hold negative views about older people. It is important that the principal practitioner and practice manager set good examples to others in the dental team to improve the chances that ageist attitudes are not revealed or acted upon.

The first signs of disability may be observed in patients aged over 50 years, and after the age of 70 years they rise steeply. According to statistics, almost 70% of disabled adults are aged 60 and over. Commonly reported disabilities in this age group are impaired mobility and hearing loss. Although the most severely affected older people tend to live in residential care, for others fears about living alone have resulted in sheltered accommodation for older people. Dentists will care for and treat a range of older people – some still living at home, others with mild disability living in sheltered accommodation and others with severe disability looked after in residential care. The requirement for dentists to be able to adjust their communication styles and skills to provide empathetic care for older people is essential.

In order to communicate effectively and be empathetic with older people, dentists must be aware of the physical health and oral treatment needs of the patient. Certain physical aids (for example, waiting areas suitable for the older patient) may make older people feel more welcome while promoting their sense of well-being when they visit the practice. The dental team should ensure that it has large-size information leaflets, magazines focused on interests of the older person, reminders to attend, individualised instructions for maintaining oral hygiene with dentures and natural teeth, special treatments for patients over 60 to retain function and appearance of dentition and prevention of late-onset caries and periodontal disease and targeting screening of oral cancer in high-risk groups (smokers over the age of 50). Some aspects of growing old involve the senses and are features that can impair communication:

- Hearing
  - one third may have hearing difficulties
  - thirty per cent are deaf in one ear
  - impairment of hearing frequencies above 4000hz is common (presbycusis)
  - inability to comprehend speech (300 to 2000hz) can also be a feature
  - tinnitus or ringing in the ears is also frequent.

- Vision
  - decline in accommodation (ability to focus)
  - cataracts, (approximately half of those aged 65 and older have a cataract)
  - alteration in colour and distance or depth perception.

Communication difficulties can therefore occur simply due to these sensory deficits not being recognised by dentists. Nevertheless for older or younger people with sensory impairments barriers to accessing health care are a consequence of inappropriate communication formats used by dentists. Dentists and their teams need to be aware of the limitations of their communication formats and the importance of in-service training in alternative communication skills.

Hearing impairment
It is recommended that members of the dental team should remove masks while communicating, attempt to reduce the impact of 'dental noise', to have knowledge of basic sign language and to use alternative communication methods, such as Makaton©.

People with a hearing impairment attending for dental care may range from those with tinnitus to those with profound hearing loss. Dentists should provide facilities that will enable them to communicate effectively with people with a hearing impairment. It has been suggested that someone in the practice should have signing skills and act as a sign-language interpreter for patients with hearing impairment.

Taking a full medical history can be a challenge with a patient with deafness. Patients with a gradual developing hearing impairment adapt and compensate by lip-reading. Therefore the dental practitioner should:
- lower or remove a face mask when conversing with the patient
- sit directly opposite [to face] the patient
- speak normally but at a somewhat slower pace
- stop frequently to allow the patient to ask for clarification
- sit away from a bright background (for example, sunlight through a window) to avoid casting a shadow on his/her face
- use pencil and paper to assist with communications and remind patient of instructions given for self-care outside of surgery
- avoid background noises with patients using a hearing aid
- encourage patients to switch off the hearing aid prior to use of high-speed drill and other high pitched devices such as scaling devices.

Visual impairment
People with visual impairments have commented upon their lack of enthusiasm to care for their oral health. This has been related to feelings of low-spiritedness and depression associated with the loss of sight. There is a need for members of the dental team to provide dental health information in a manner that has meaning for people who have lost their sight. Touch has been used as a medium to increase awareness of dental health in visually impaired children and adolescents. The 'Tooth Touch Kit' was developed to explain treatment and to provide information for promoting dental health. More recently, attitudes of dental health professionals towards orthodontic care for the visually impaired has also been investigated. The findings showed that access to orthodontic services was influenced by patient gender, onset of visual impairment and the patient-dentist perception of treatment need.

The Royal National Institute for the Blind (RNIB) has suggested that it is essential for people with sight loss to be able to make informed decisions. People with visual impairments need to access information readily so that they can give their informed consent. The RNIB suggests that written communications should be available in large print, audiotape or in Braille. 'See it Right' is a package containing practical advice on planning, designing and producing information pamphlets, which may be downloaded from the RNIB website (http://rnib.org.uk).

Communicating with People with Learning Disabilities

Communicating with people who have a learning disability must be individualistic and tailored to the needs of the person. Many people with learning disability are negativistic, perseverate and have low self-esteem. It is important for the dental team to acknowledge these characteristics and to assist the patient to accept dental care. Some people will be able to voice their treatment wishes and ask questions prior to treatment, others may need a carer to act as an interpreter within a triangular relationship with the dental healthcare professional.

For people able to articulate their wishes the relationship with the dental health professional can be invaluable. These relationships promote empowerment while enabling the individual to develop new lifestyle skills – communication, social and healthcare skills. In the following example a triangular relationship existed between the dentist, patient and carer. In this the individual with learning disability was the focal point of the communication network. Visits to the dentist allowed new relationships to be developed, while the carer acted as translator, enabling the communications between dentist and patient to be acted upon. The mother of a 55-year-old man with mild learning disability stated: 'John enjoys his visits to Mr Smith's surgery. He doesn't listen to me about brushing his teeth. If I ask him to do it he doesn't, but if Mr Smith speaks to John about brushing his teeth or not eating so many sweets John tries to be compliant. So when John doesn't want to brush his teeth, I say: 'Mr Smith would like you to, and remember how he said it was good for your teeth', and John says 'Well, alright then'. I like to think of it as a triangle that I'm part of. Mr Smith takes time putting the information over carefully to John. He repeats it in a very deliberate way. I think the best things about John's visits are that John talks to Mr Smith and his nurse and that I'm not there.'

Carers are important allies in treatment situations where language skills are less developed. The clinical vignette of a woman dentist treating an 11-year-old boy with Asperger's syndrome is illustrative. It shows how the parents/carers, as a result of their closeness with the individual with learning disability, can act as a communication interpreter: 'At the start, Jimmy's lack of eye contact made it hard and he made a lot of noise during the treatment.

As time went on I started to understand that Jimmy was communicating with me. I realised it when I gave him an ID block. I asked him if he was numb, and Jimmy said: 'Chickenpox!' I didn't understand but his mother said: 'Jimmy had chickenpox in the summer and he was itchy.' From then on I knew that 'chickenpox' meant he was going numb. I needed the mother as translator.'

Research has shown that the inclusion of parents/carers within the communication network is important when providing care for young adults with a profound learning disability. Parents were able to identify when their children were experiencing 'new pains'. They were aware of their children exhibiting new and unusual behaviours. They saw their children withdrawing, crying or moaning, odd facial expressions, grinding their teeth, head banging or changes in postures. The integration of parents' knowledge of their children's behaviours allowed parents to build up a checklist. When they observed the behaviours on the 'pain checklist' they would organise medical or dental care. The inclusion of parents/carers in the communication process is therefore essential. Dentists must use parents'/carers' knowledge of their children's needs and incorporate this information into their treatment and patient management strategies.

Dentists must use verbal and written communications that reflect the patient's age and degree of understanding. Appropriate uncomplicated and non-technical (non-jargon) language should be used. MENCAP has suggested using a technique called 'jargon buster' to promote the use of plain English. Jargon-busting is using simple words to explain more complicated concepts – for example, using 'about' instead of 'concerning' or 'soon' instead of 'in the near future'. This is of particular significance when written information is presented to the patient with a learning disability.

Issues surrounding consent have been discussed elsewhere, but it is worth emphasising that the need to obtain consent from children and adults with a learning disability is mandatory. In such clinical situations, it is important that written material is easily understood and that the patient gives informed consent. MENCAP has written a series of pamphlets concerned with health and other issues pertaining to the lives of those with learning disability. These may be obtained from the MENCAP website (www.mencap.com) and are examples of materials written specifically for those with a learning disability.

Other communication systems exist, and these are used in a variety of settings for people with communication difficulties. Examples of these alter-

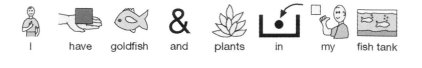

| I | have | goldfish | and | plants | in | my | fish tank |

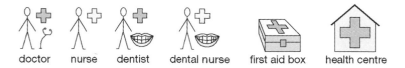

| doctor | nurse | dentist | dental nurse | first aid box | health centre |

Fig 4-1 Writing with symbols 2000© Widget Software.

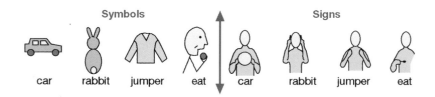

Symbols   Signs

| car | rabbit | jumper | eat | car | rabbit | jumper | eat |

Fig 4-2 Examples of Makaton Vocabulary©.

native approaches are the Wigit© 'Writing with Symbols' (Fig 4-1) and the Makaton Vocabulary© (Fig 4-2).

Makaton© was developed in the 1970s for children and adults with communication difficulties. It uses both signs and symbols to help children and adults communicate effectively with dental health professionals. Makaton© has been used in many different settings, including the dental surgery. Home-first Community Trust in Ballymena, Northern Ireland, has published *Going to the Dentist*. This book has been designed to be used with or without assistance. It describes a number of different dental healthcare skills and dental treatments, such as extractions, radiographs and fillings. It also includes a section on gaining consent.

MENCAP has provided a checklist of good practice in its policy document *Am I Making Myself Clear?*:

- Plan what you want to say: cut out unnecessary detail and present information in a simple, step-by-step way.
- Try to write as you speak: do not use jargon, use simple words to explain complicated points.
- Keep sentences short.
- use active and personal language: use 'you' and 'we', as this is direct and understandable.
- Use numbers and not words – examples given by MENCAP include 'use 3 instead of three' and 'many' instead of '1,000'.
- Make it clear what action has to be taken: symbols should be included, and the symbols should support the text.
- The use of drawings or photographs may link pieces of information together.
- Use a font size of greater than 14 for ease of reading.

Communicating with People with Mental Illness

Patients with mental illness tend to receive less dental treatment, which may be of a lower quality compared with the general population. As a group people with mental illness may be vulnerable to oral health problems. The relatively poor dental health of psychiatric patients is characterised by missing and discoloured teeth, periodontal disease and halitosis. In addition, many antipsychotic drugs can cause a dry mouth, resulting in oral discomfort and increased experience of dental caries. Recent work examining the dental health of psychiatric patients showed that many oral health needs among such patients were a result of:

- frequent and large consumption of non-milk extrinsic sugars
- lack of oral hygiene and use of fluoride toothpaste
- medication causing a dry mouth, reducing the protective effect of saliva and associated increase in dental caries
- cigarette smoking, compounded by the lack of a filter in 'rollup' cigarettes, leading to tobacco-induced oral mucosal conditions.

To address these patients' oral health problems collaborative approaches to their dental care must be instigated between all healthcare providers. They may do this by communicating with general medical practitioners and psychiatric carers to ensure that these patients have equitable access to treatment and services.

Communicating with People from Ethnic Minorities

When considering the dental health needs of ethnic minority groups communication difficulties arise because English may be a second language and the meaning of illness, the expression of symptoms and treatment may be different from those expressed by the indigenous population.

Specific difficulties are considered to be associated with health professionals' misunderstandings of the presentation of symptoms – for example, expressions of pain - the meaning of the symptom for the patient and compliance with the treatment regime - for example, fear of bleeding, as this will sap away vital energy. In order to overcome these difficulties, it has been suggested that there is a need for health professionals to improve their awareness of the meanings of illness and develop their communication skills. It has been suggested that clinicians should acquire a knowledge of the 'language of distress', avoid jargon and attempt to explain the symptoms and treatment in lay terms. This has particular relevance for dental care of Chinese people. It has been shown that costs, language and communication problems as well as fears about the treatment have resulted in barriers to dental attendance. Various suggestions have been made to reduce barriers to dental attendance for Chinese people. These include:
- improving dental personnel's cultural proficiency through training
- dental services provided by ethnic minority groups
- interpreting and advocacy services
- culturally and linguistically appropriate dental health information services.

Communicating with the Homeless Patient

The chaotic lifestyle of many homeless people may mean that they will attend for dental care in an emergency. The oral health needs of homeless people are known to be acute and to cause discomfort and pain. The barriers to dental care have been classified as belonging to the patient, the dentist and the dental healthcare system. Recommendations for the oral healthcare provision for homeless people have suggested that all sectors of dentistry should be involved in the care of this vulnerable group of patients.

Conclusions

The aim of this chapter was to define what is meant by the phrase 'special needs' and to provide practitioners with examples of how they may modify their communication skills to care for and promote the oral health of patients with special needs. Various alternative communication formats are suggested.

Further Reading

MAKATON – www.makaton.org

Royal National Institute for the Blind – www.rnib.org.uk

MENCAP – www.mencap.com

British Dental Association. Oral Healthcare for Older People: 2020 Vision. London: BDA, 2003.

British Dental Association. Caring for Older People's Teeth. London: BDA, 2003.

British Dental Association. Dental Care for Homeless People. London: BDA Policy Discussion Paper, 2003.

Chapter 5

Understanding and Finding Solutions: The Dentally Anxious Patient

Aim

To outline the development of dental anxiety, its assessment and management in adult dental services.

Outcome

The reader will be able to explain the major factors responsible for patients becoming dentally anxious. In addition the reader will be able to state various methods of assessing dental anxiety. Finally, the reader will be conversant with a number of behavioural management techniques for the dentally anxious patient.

Dental Anxiety: A Perpetual Problem?

It is not an exaggeration to argue that dental anxiety is the most important psychological factor dental staff will meet in practice. Dental anxiety is that feeling of apprehension experienced by an individual when confronted with matters that are dentally related. It is commonly described as having physiological, cognitive and behavioural aspects. Hence, patients who describe themselves as dentally anxious may complain of raised heart rate (physiological), imagining painful consequences of dental treatment (cognitive) and preferring to delay making a dental appointment (behavioural).

The prevalence of dental anxiety has been studied over the past 50 years. Levels of self-reported dental anxiety appear to be remarkably stable when comparing representative samples from a single culture (USA) over a time span of 34 years (1967-2001) and using identical measures (Corah's Dental Anxiety Scale). This may appear to be disappointing, especially when attempts are being made to make dental treatment more comfortable. Repeated surveys in the UK, however, suggest that dental anxiety prevalence has fallen due to procedures that have assisted in reducing anxiety. These include use of preventive treatments, lasers, new dental materials for fixing restorations, and use of written and computer-assisted information systems. The falling levels of dental anxiety may be something of a success story for the dental profession, considering there has been a definite rise of general anxiety levels in the population over the past 50 years.

From this optimistic standpoint, it is still disappointing that approximately 30% of the adult population continue to feel nervous about visiting the dentist. In a large Dutch representative sample it was found that 36% of respondents 'dreaded' visiting the dentist. Hence nervousness may not seem too important until it is realised that about one in five respondents delay making a dental appointment because of their anxiety. Dental anxiety promotes avoidance. So ubiquitous is the 'condition' of dental anxiety that the experienced practitioner with large numbers of patients, many of whom will be dentally anxious, is able to manage the vast majority of patients with quick and simple procedures that are learnt from observing or copying other colleagues, training courses and general clinical experience. Some patients present, however, with either unusual features that may not respond quickly to the dental practitioner's standard procedure or with such intensity that at first sight the anxiety cannot be challenged in order to diminish it. This group are sometimes classified, rather punitively, as 'difficult' patients. The term indicates that their treatment cannot be delivered in the normal way but special procedures are indicated. However, 'difficult' could be interpreted to mean that the patient has a choice over whether to volunteer his/her feelings. S/he might have made a hedonistic decision to receive special attention and extra time from the dental team. Evidence would appear to indicate the reverse. Most dentally anxious patients are acutely embarrassed to admit to their difficulty and would gladly prefer, if at all possible, to hide their feelings and attempt to cope without any special arrangements and procedures. The more intense the quality and quantity of anxiety felt by the patient, the greater the sense of shame and need to avoid any exposure to the dentist or dentally related stimuli. Therefore a distinction needs to be made between those patients who attend despite of their intense fear (dentally anxious) and those who avoid dental treatment (dentally phobic).

Individuals who avoid dental care at all costs are best described as dentally phobic, which is distinct and separate from dental anxiety. While dentally anxious patients can link their fear to specific frightening dental experiences, the same is not the case for those who are dentally phobic. Dentally phobic patients tend to displace or foist frightening experiences from outside the dental surgery onto dental treatment. The resulting anxiety is unbearable, and they avoid the situation that evokes such a magnitude of fear – that is dental treatment. Therefore dental phobia is a condition with discrete fea-

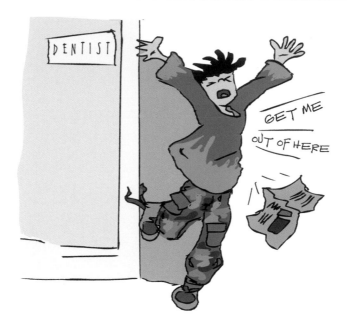

tures, which can be a symptom of a psychological disorder and as such may require referral for secondary-level care.

Dental anxiety develops in a variety of ways as follows:
- a direct traumatic dental experience, such as a painful injection or exposure to insensitive dental staff
- an indirect traumatic dental experience, such as hearing negative stories about dental procedures in the family, school playground or articles in magazines, books and the media
- a direct traumatic medical experience, such as lumbar puncture or tonsillectomy conducted at an early age.

These various traumatic experiences are interpreted by the individual under a number of conditions that have a bearing on the strength and stability of dental anxiety, including:
- the vulnerability of the individual concerned. Patients with multiple mental health problems or a generally anxious disposition may be more prone to developing dental anxiety
- the timing of the experience. Patients who encounter a dental (or perhaps medically-related) traumatic experience at an early age (under five years of age) are more likely to exhibit dental anxiety

- the frequency and intensity of the dental traumatic experience. Repeated unpleasant experiences or a single very intense experience (dental or medical) may be foisted or displaced upon the dental situation and generate profound dental anxiety
- the sequence of events. If the first visit to the dentist by a child patient is frightening and traumatic then the chances of dental anxiety developing is significantly greater compared to a child who has had a number of pleasant experiences prior to an unpleasant, say painful, experience. The coping abilities of the patient to help the child and for the experience to be labelled as non-threatening is partially dependent on reviewing the wider motives for visiting the dentist (maintaining dental health) and the attitudes of the dental team (sensitive and caring staff).

Dental anxiety is reported more strongly in women than men, in younger rather than older people and in those with greater untreated dental disease. People who are dentally anxious tend not to have an extensive past dental treatment history, as shown by a limited number of filled tooth surfaces but more teeth missing for non-orthodontic reasons. Surprisingly, dental anxiety does not necessarily decrease when all teeth are lost. There is some evidence that amongst the edentulous there is a greater proportion of very anxious people compared with the dentate. This may be due to patients who have been very dentally anxious at a younger age, opting to have a clearance to reduce the need to visit the dentist. Their dental anxiety remains high. The expected relief from dental anxiety for this anxious group does not occur, as they do not need to challenge their anxiety any longer and cannot find reassurance that might have been possible from successful treatment visits. Dentally anxious patients are more likely to state they are experiencing dental symptoms such as sore gums, toothache and bad breath. The explanation of this effect is probably not straightforward. A dentally anxious person may avoid the dentist and delay attention, thereby allowing disease levels to increase. Alternatively, these patients may be generally more concerned about their well-being and volunteer their problems more readily. Another clear feature of patients with high levels of dental anxiety is that their pain tolerance threshold is reduced. The dental practitioner therefore needs to offer local anaesthesia to dentally anxious patients whenever there is a small chance of sensations due to a treatment intervention becoming uncomfortable. Of course the administration of local anaesthesia for some dentally anxious patients is a challenge in itself.

Not all patients develop dental anxiety in their childhood years. Longitudinal studies have shown that young adults (18-26) can develop dental anxi-

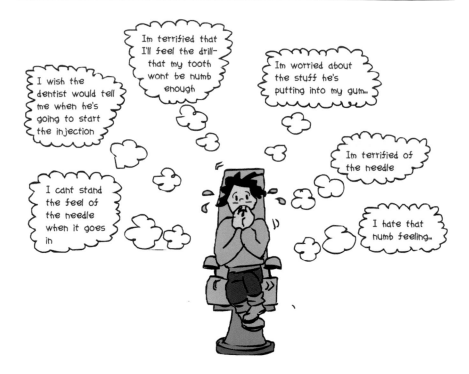

ety (incidence of becoming anxious greater than 10%). Factors that predict the development of dental anxiety among this age group include patchy dental attendance, aversive experience, such as pain, or the extraction of one or more teeth, and multiple fears.

Assessment of Dental Anxiety

For practical purposes the best methods of assessing dental anxiety include observation and asking the patient directly. Observational methods adopted routinely by the dental practitioner can be efficient and assist when patients are attempting to put a brave face on anticipated pain. The later method can be employed by a direct question such as 'how do you feel about coming to the dentist?' or by a series of questions that can be formally presented by means of a questionnaire.

There are advantages to using standardised dental anxiety questionnaires (see Table 5-1). The dental practitioner who uses these questionnaires routinely will become more familiar with interpreting the scores obtained and can

39

Table 5-1 **Advantages and disadvantages of using standardised dental anxiety questionnaires**

Advantages
Identifies if a particular procedure was anxiety-provoking
Acts as a focused vehicle for more detailed discussion and assessment
Enables a permanent record to appear in the patient notes
Alerts colleagues in practice to patients' anxieties on return visits
Reduces anxiety in patients (short-term effect)

Disadvantages
Some patients reluctant to complete
Time for patient to complete
Cost of printing
Extra administration

develop how to use them in collaboration with the patient. There are few contraindications to using these questionnaires. Some patients may prefer not to complete the pro-formas and are ashamed to admit high levels of anxiety. Some sensitive questioning to ascertain these reasons may be particularly fruitful in helping to understand these patients' difficulties in attending the dentist. However, the wishes of patients should be respected if they prefer their comments and ratings not to be logged. Time is required for the questionnaires to be completed, and there is a small print cost. However, completion, in most cases, can be organised in the waiting room by the receptionists. An advantage of using the questionnaires in this manner is that patients may be reassured by handing their reply to the dentist. The expectation that the dentist is aware of their feelings as recorded on paper may be sufficient to allow treatments to be achieved more smoothly.

In-depth interviews with patients with profound dental anxiety have shown that patients valued tremendously the dentist remembering their particular concerns about attending and treatment fears. In addition, recent work has revealed the importance of practitioners taking a positive and broad holistic approach with these patients. Dentists who are able to demonstrate to their anxious patients that they are trustworthy will be more successful in completing treatments. The implication for the practitioner that s/he may not be trustworthy can be an unpleasant realisation when treating dentally anxious patients. The important point to stress is that the patient will harbour negative stereotypical beliefs (dentists are uncaring, and so on) that the dentist can modify. Hence, appropriate facial expressions (smiling, use of eye contact, and so on) and openness and sensitivity in communication style can be important signals, indicating safety to the patient. Furthermore, ensuring that the patient has a means of indicating his/her distress about the dental visit will incrementally, over time, improve patient confidence and abate fears.

Behavioural Management and Dental Anxiety

Effective communication and history-taking forms the first part of the psychological management of the dentally anxious patient. In a non-clinical setting the dentist establishes rapport with the patient, allows him/her to express anxieties, relate previous experiences and discuss his/her oral health status and treatment possibilities. The dentist can explain the various options available to obtain dental fitness and rehearse with the patient the strategies to encourage acceptance of the procedures necessary. For example, patients with a moderate anxiety towards needles may agree to have a local anaesthetic if the dentist gives them the opportunity to say what aspect of the injection procedure they find unpleasant - the initial insertion of the needle, the lack of forewarning of the impending puncture, the sensation of the anaesthetic agent, the consequence of the numbing effect, worry associated with whether the tooth will be completely numb and so on.

Some patients welcome a detailed explanation of the procedures to be used in treatment. This can be best demonstrated by a running commentary at each stage of the treatment. However, the dental practitioner should check with patients if they are the sort of person who prefers detailed information or likes the dentist to simply proceed and allow them to distract themselves from the situation. It is hard to generalise which type of individuals prefer to 'monitor' what is going on and those who choose to ignore their surroundings as much as possible. Some estimates put the proportion of the latter as about 10%. Again, the importance of trying not to generalise about anxious patients must be stressed. Individual approaches to assessment and treatment are therefore indicated.

With more severe cases simply discussing the difficulty may be insufficient, and some preparatory procedures may be required. These may be termed systematic desensitisation techniques and rely on the patient being coaxed along a hierarchy of progressively more difficult situations. Speedy progress can be made if the rationale of the procedure is explained and a key element is adhered to – that is, patients are assured that, should they wish to break off their attempt to tolerate the next procedure along the hierarchy and pause, they are free to do so. With gentle encouragement the patient progresses along the hierarchy to confront each step up to the goal of receiving the local anaesthetic. The patient is praised at each step for his/her 'success'. Should this process take longer than a single session it is important for the practitioner to remember the last step reached and maybe backtrack to build up the patient's confidence of the newly developed tolerance. Instructing patients to indicate if they want to withdraw at any time and giving clear instructions about what is about to happen will increase the sense of trust. Effective communication is a vital part of non-pharmacological techniques, such as 'tell-show-do', desensitising hierarchy, relaxation and hypnosis.

Tell-Show-Do

This is a simple means of preparing children and anxious adults for dental care. The dentist tells the patient what is to be completed, shows the patient what will be done and then does it. The ability of the dentist to use language the patient can understand assists in reducing anticipatory fears. A simple tell-show-do scenario prior to general anaesthesia can reduce dental anxiety and heart rate prior to the extraction of teeth.

Other techniques can be applied to reduce anxiety, and their underlying principles vary. These procedures have been applied with some success but are dependent on the practitioner making an investment in time, interest and in some cases specialist equipment (for example, heart-rate monitors in the case of biofeedback).

Hypnosis

This procedure is based on switching the patient's attention to some external object or an internal bodily stimulus that is unrelated to dentistry. The aim is to alter the patient's state of consciousness to induce a sense of mus-

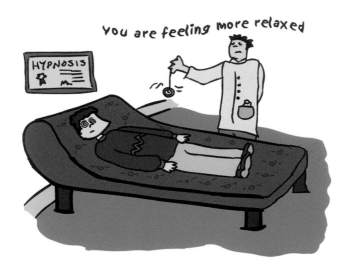

cular relaxation and is assisted by a high level of suggestibility within the patient. Hypnosis has been used widely in dentistry to attenuate anxiety and induce states of relaxation. A disadvantage of hypnosis is that with increased anxiety it is harder for the patient to relax and enter the hypnotic state. Practitioners with an interest in hypnosis can obtain local support and training from the British Society of Medical and Dental Hypnosis (www.bsmdh.org) and the International Society of Hypnosis, which has its central offices in Melbourne, Australia (www.ish.unimelb.edu.au).

Biofeedback

This procedure trains patients to recognise their physiological responses by reference to a variable scale presented visually (for example, a meter) or audibly (for example, a tone). Typically the physiological response to dental procedures, or other anxiety-provoking situations in the dental surgery, produces a raised level on the chosen measure. The technique assumes that individuals who monitor themselves with very accurate information about their physiological processes can gain a form of voluntary mastery over what has been traditionally understood as involuntary processes. Biofeedback has been used with some effect in the dental environment, but has probably been superseded by verbal techniques not requiring specialist equipment. The advent of new miniaturised transducers of physiological indicators, such as heart rate monitors on a wristwatch device, may signal an upsurge of interest in these procedures.

Relaxation

The general principle behind relaxation is that a relaxed state cannot co-exist with anxiety. This has led some theorists to recognise relaxation as inhibitory of anxiety. Although relaxation is not an essential requisite for anxiety reduction, as methods exposing the patient to feared objects such as needles can produce results without the patient being relaxed, it is generally beneficial. It is recognised that the pain tolerance threshold is raised when an individual is relaxed, hence it is a worthwhile state to encourage in the dental surgery. A popular technique for dentally anxious patients will be to instruct them to tense and then relax systematically specific sets of muscles throughout the body. This procedure can be demonstrated in a single appointment by taking patients through the exercise, which would require about 15-20 minutes. An audiotape of the procedure adopted within the practice can then be handed to the patient to practise at home in preparation for the next appointment. With practice the patient can quickly run through the relaxation exercise in the dental chair to obtain a general feeling of relaxation and well-being in readiness for dental treatment. There are various methods to support the patient to achieve a good level of relaxation, mainly environmental in nature, such as quiet surroundings, selection of music offered, pleasant pictures on walls or ceiling, and a generally unhurried manner from the staff - that is, no sudden movements or exclamations.

Long-Term Follow-up and Continuing Care

Once dentally anxious patients have successfully received treatment the dental practitioner can assist them further to maintain their ability to receive dental treatment. Some practical points practitioners can adopt for their practice include:

- Praise patients for undergoing the treatment they were fearful of. Make reference to the considerable achievement that has been made by inviting them to remember the extent of their fear prior to the treatment.
- Restate that the treatment they have received will have improved their dental health status and eliminate the need for more extensive treatment.
- Ensure that patients are reminded that the methods they used to help themselves through the procedures will work again. This will assist with the development of self-efficacy, that is their own sense of confidence of coping with their anxious feelings. Patients whose confidence in their abilities to tolerate anxiety has been increased are known to be more successful in completing treatment.

- Place a reference to their particular anxiety in the dental notes (for example, 'anxious about injection') and remind patients on revisit, should treatment again be necessary, that they prefer to have this approach to assist with treatment. Research with dentally anxious patients has shown that confidence in the dentist is retained if the dental team is able to reassure patients of the success of previous techniques.
- Do not assume that dentally anxious patients will 'get over' their anxiety with time. Unfortunately, dental anxiety is remarkably stable and, rather than diminish over time, may well increase in some individuals.
- Patients are to be encouraged to visit regularly for check-up appointments to help them become used to the dental environment and the personnel. The longer the interval between each visit, the more likely it is that their anxiety will return to pre-treatment levels.
- A long-term approach will be required, and patients may need many years of active clinical assistance before their anxiety can be said to have receded to insignificance. Whereas dental anxiety is known to decrease with age, this evidence has been gleaned mainly from cross-sectional studies where cohort effects (separate age groups, each with their own collected experience of dental treatment) have not been removed. Individuals may not demonstrate the advantages of simply increasing years but carry with them memories of their dental treatment history. The dental practitioner should not take for granted that the patient's anxiety can be ignored purely as a factor of the number of years that have passed. Rather, the patient will be thankful for being treated with such thoughtfulness.
- If at any stage the dental practitioner is unsure of the patient's response to a particular procedure or treatment plan, an open-ended question can be adopted, such as 'How do you feel about …?' to check the patient's possible response.
- Judicious use of minimal interventive dental techniques, thereby avoiding overambitious care – for example, employing shortened dental arch therapy in older patients to obviate the need to attempt complex, stressful/challenging care of permanent molars.

Conclusions

The reward of successfully treating the dentally anxious patient can be determined by the extent to which the patient makes subsequent visits. The practitioner can achieve considerable progress with a thorough understanding of the area of dental anxiety and methods of anxiety management. Severe cases of dental anxiety, which can be referred to as dental phobia, are very infrequent visitors to the dentist. It is likely that the dental phobic will attend the dentist only when in great discomfort or following trauma, and the chances of achieving rapid resolution of the problem is low when resorting to behavioural management procedures. In extreme cases of dental anxiety, psychotherapeutic interventions may be indicated from suitably qualified clinicians. The use of standard approaches outlined in this chapter should enable the practitioner to provide routine dental care, and therefore enable the anxious patient to visit the dentist without fear. Attention to the patient's feelings about visits at future appointments will maintain the positive response to the dentist.

Further Reading

Burke FJT, Freeman R. Preparing for Dental Practice. Oxford: Oxford University Press, 2004.

Elmore AM. Biofeedback therapy in the treatment of dental anxiety and dental phobia. Dental Clinics of North America 1998;32:(4)735-744.

Humphris GM, Ling M. Behavioural Sciences for Dentistry. Edinburgh: Churchill Livingstone, 2000.

Chapter 6

Understanding and Finding Solutions: The 'Difficult' and Dissatisfied Patient

Aim

The aim of this chapter is to provide the reader with an understanding of patients with difficulties, how they disrupt the treatment relationship with the dentist (the treatment alliance) and to consider some management solutions and treatment decisions.

Outcome

At the end of this chapter the reader should understand why some patients appear to act in a difficult way, a means by which you may discover the source of their difficulties, what is meant by the treatment alliance and a decision-making framework with regard to their management.

Defining Difficult Patients

Essentially, difficult patients are patients who experience difficulties. For some patients these difficulties are external and are often current life problems (for example, recent divorce). These patients shift or displace their current problems onto dental treatment. For other patients internal or psychological difficulties are shifted onto dentistry. Difficulties may present as oral symptoms (for example, burning tongue) or physical symptoms (for example, altered perception of appearance). A third category of difficult patients exists – those who present with oral manifestations of certain physical illnesses. While patients who present with psychological or physical illness may remain in the care of their dentists, treatment must proceed with caution. It may be appropriate for these patients to be referred to their GPs. Dentists have an important role in patient management, as they may be the first to recognise a patient with emotional difficulties or certain illnesses.

The three clinical vignettes that follow are illustrative. In the first case a woman patient with phantom toothache displaced her unhappiness and malcontent associated with divorcing her husband after a long separation onto her mouth. In the second case a young woman presenting with dysmorphophobic symptoms displaced her anxieties onto the appearance of her teeth. In the final case a 50-year-old man complained of a dry and painful mouth associated with lethargy and depression.

Vignette 1: A Case of Phantom Toothache

A woman attended a dental practice for treatment. She had toothache and demanded that her teeth be root-treated. She returned some months later to demand that the dentist extract the root-filled teeth. Her medical history was remarkable, as in the past five years she had been hospitalised for an appendectomy, hysterectomy and cholecystectomy.

The patient was 40-years-old, recently divorced and lived with her elderly parents. She had been separated from her husband for five years. She complained about the pain of her personal circumstances and felt lost without her husband. It occurred to the dentist that the complaints about the physical pains – in her abdomen and in her teeth – started soon after he left. She could see little relevance between her life experiences and her current predicament, but the dentist's comment and concern afforded her some symptomatic relief as the pain in her teeth subsided. As the pain diminished the dentist and the practice staff were harangued with a series of complaints about how she had been treated. The mention or the sight of her name in the appointment book resulted in sinking spirits. Nevertheless, despite the patient's complaints she was grateful to the dentist and his staff. She remains with the practice to this day.

Vignette 2: A Case of Dysmorphophobia

Dysmorphophobia is 'a subjective feeling of ugliness or physical defect that the patient feels is noticeable to others, although his/her appearance is within normal limits'. The choice of symptom varies, with many different parts of the body being 'chosen'. They include the teeth, nose, breath, shape of face, genitalia and so on. Dysmorphophobia is the presenting symptom. The underlying psychopathology may range from current life difficulties to mental health problems. In late adolescence or early adulthood it may be prodromal of schizophrenia. When the choice of symptom is the teeth, breath or shape of face the dentist may be the first to identify patients with dysmorphophobia. The referral of such patients to their GPs for psychiatric assessment is essential.

A 23-year-old single woman was referred to a university department of restorative dentistry because of her inappropriate reaction to anterior crowns. The crowns had been provided twice and the patient was distressed by their appearance. She insisted that her teeth looked ugly and her mouth was 'dirty and freak-like'. She refused to go out, and if anyone came to the door she would hide. She became a virtual recluse. As a child the patient had traumatised a deciduous central incisor, causing injury to her lips. It also caused delayed eruption of the permanent successor. She considered the permanent tooth 'ugly and freak-like'. The patient became very self-conscious about her teeth and their appearance. Her father was an aggressive alcoholic. As a child, the patient had observed many violent arguments between her parents, during which her mother would be hit in the mouth, damaging her lips and teeth. The patient had been traumatised by these events. She had shifted her anxieties of her mother's mouth injuries to her own injuries as a child (trauma to her own lips and teeth) and to the crowns (perceived as damaged teeth).

Vignette 3: A Man with a Dry and Painful Mouth

A 50-year-old man complained bitterly about his doctor who refused to treat him. Mr T was venomous in his verbal attack on the medical practitioner and was now without a doctor. His mouth was very painful and dry, and he complained of tiredness and lack of energy. He felt 'depressed'. The dentist knew of the patient's family circumstances and the decision to sell the family business, which resulted in his taking early retirement. The dentist assumed that the patient's depression was associated with the loss of his business. He also thought that the dry mouth was related to his depressive state, but he was concerned about the lethargy. As the patient was without a doctor, the dentist referred him to the local hospital for examination. At his routine check-up appointment the patient voiced his gratitude to his dentist. As a result of his hospital appointment he had been diagnosed with diabetes. He felt he had been cared for, and on the advice of a relative had found a new medical practitioner.

Considering these cases, it is possible to expand the definition of 'difficult' patients. 'Difficult' patients are patients who experience difficulties in their current lives, they tend to be anxious and through a process of displacement onto dental matters they tend to make their difficulties the problems of the dental surgery. In some instances patients who present with difficulties are suffering from physical illness. These patients must be referred for medical assessment, as in the third vignette. Therefore, irrespective of the sources of their difficulties (external or internal) they can cause considerable problems for those involved in the provision of their dental care.

The Dentist-Patient Relationship and the Treatment Alliance

Issues surrounding patient management are at the centre of the difficulties patients perpetuate for those in the dental team caring for their treatment. The patients' complaints, disagreeableness and anxieties can be so great as to upset the dentist-patient relationship. There are three aspects to the dentist-patient relationship: first, the real relationship, which is an adult-to-adult interaction, based on the reality of the dentist's expertise; secondly, the treatment alliance, which is the kernel of the dentist-patient relationship and, thirdly, the transference, which is an adult (dentist)-to-child (patient) relationship in which the patient's previous important relationships and associated feelings are foisted (displaced) onto the dentist.

The treatment alliance may be defined as a two-person (adult) endeavour, with dentist and the patient working together towards a common treatment goal. The dentist must monitor the patients' needs while assessing his/her own responses to the patient's demands. The dentist paves the patient's way to accept the dental treatment being offered and provided. The treatment alliance reflects the real relationship, positive aspects of the dentist-patient encounter and a containment of anxieties and worries on the part of the patient and of the dentist. Essentially, the treatment alliance reflects a balanced interaction based on good communication and understanding. This helps to reduce occupational stress in the dental team by facilitating clinical practice.

How can the treatment alliance assist in understanding the problems experienced by dentists when treating patients with difficulties? It is suggested that the complaints, anxieties and disagreeableness displaced from external and current life problems, or the emotional difficulties displaced from internal, psychological problems, serve to disrupt the treatment alliance. In such situations it is impossible for the patient's difficulties to be contained and there is a breakdown in the dentist-patient relationship. It is possible to conceptualise the breakdown in terms of transference, but it is more helpful to think of it in terms of the treatment alliance and, as a consequence, of poor communication and understanding.

The ability of the dentist to restore the treatment alliance is important. The dentist needs to make the decision as to whether (s)he has the appropriate skills to do so. Kay and Nuttall's (1995) work in clinical decision-making is essential reading. In their clinical decision-making framework (Fig 6-1) Kay and Nuttall list the various clinical and communication skills necessary when coming to the decision to provide dental treatment for patients.

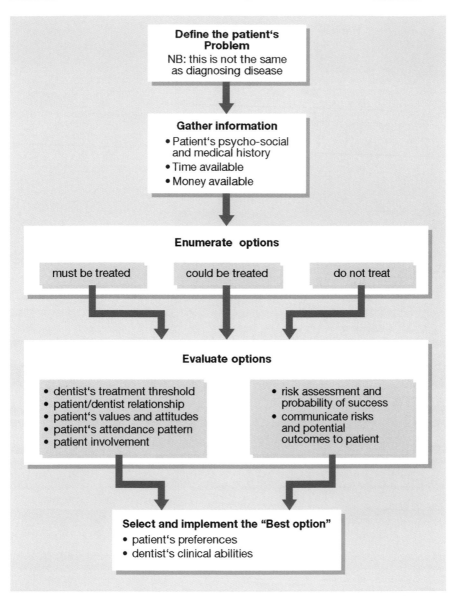

Fig 6-1 Rational decision-making. Reprinted with kind permission of the BDJ. Kay E, Nuttall N. Clinical decision making-an art or a science? Part V: Patient preferences and their influence on decision making British Dental Journal 1995.178 229-233.

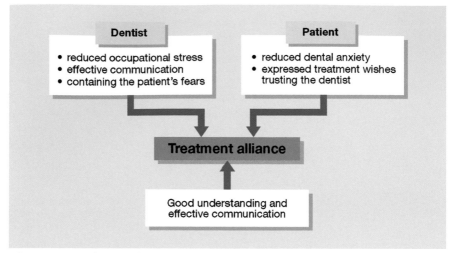

Fig 6-2 Strengthening the treatment alliance.

They insist that the dentist must find out about patients in terms of their past medical and dental histories and in terms of their life experiences and current life events. They point out the importance of what cannot be treated, what can be treated and what must be treated. They envisage dental treatment as a skills-based exercise and highlight the equality of the dentist's clinical and patient management skills. The equality of these skills reflects the dentist's ability to contain the emotional 'off-load' from patients with difficulties. The dentist's containment skills (for instance, communication skills, being able to withstand the patient's complaints) strengthens the treatment alliance. It is the key in the decision-making process to care for patients with difficulties.

Two clinical scenarios follow. In the first case a multidisciplinary approach, relying on patient collaboration, was used to maintain a treatment alliance with the patient. In the second scenario the issue of a patient with a severe and disruptive gag reflex is outlined. Recommendations to assist in management and so maintain the treatment alliance are provided.

1. The importance of considering the patient's treatment preferences has been highlighted in creating the treatment alliance. Chapple et al (2003) describe patients' preferences for a collaborative role with their dentists when decisions are being made about their treatment. The case of a 23-year-old single woman with dysmorphophobia provides an illustration of

how a multidisciplinary approach and collaborative working with the patient allowed dental treatment to be successful. The dentist was supported throughout the treatment by the patient's ongoing psychotherapy and by a supportive dental technician. There were two aspects to the patient's treatment:

- twice-weekly psychotherapeutic treatment on an open ended contract. This allowed the patient's anxieties to be aired and the source of her difficulties to be highlighted. She gradually understood that she had foisted earlier life difficulties onto the appearance of her teeth. This enabled her to accept her new crowns and to return to socialise with family and friends.
- clinical treatment: Close liaison between dentist and technician was critical. Old photographs were obtained from the patient. These allowed a diagnostic wax-up to be made of the proposed form for the replacement crowns. The existing crowns were removed and preparations modified. Provisional crowns were made using a template that had been pressure-formed from the duplicate remodelled cast. The laboratory-made provisional crowns replaced the temporary crowns. Over a period of six months these crowns were continuously modified until the patient was completely satisfied. This coincided with her realisation that her anxiety belonged to earlier times and not with the crowns. The technician meticulously copied the morphology in porcelain, including characterisation and shading, as selected by the patient. The patient was delighted. She functions well and remains happy with the appearance of her teeth.

In this case the treatment alliance was strengthened in a variety of ways. The dentist was provided with support from the patient's psychotherapeutic treatment and by the dental technician. Multidisciplinary working enabled the dentist to contain her own frustrations and reduce her occupational stress. The dentist was able to communicate effectively with the patient, understand her considerable difficulties and appreciate her fears. This allowed the dentist to work collaboratively with the patient, who was assisted throughout the treatment by her psychotherapy. This allowed her to realise the inappropriate nature of her pre-occupation with her teeth. The treatment alliance was strengthened by multidisciplinary working and the collaborative role the patient had in her treatment (Fig 6-3).

2. Patients with a pronounced and disruptive gagging reflex can disturb the treatment alliance. Their gagging reflex is so disturbing that they avoid treatment, and when they do attend they are labelled as 'difficult'. Impression-taking is a mildly unpleasant experience for most patients. However, a small but significant proportion are severely affected. Patients with disruptive gag-

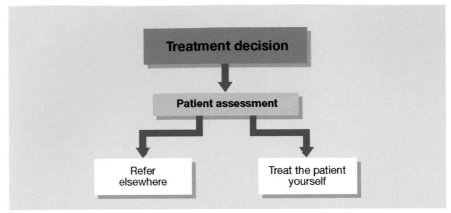

Fig 6-3 Decision-making and patient assessment.

ging have been described as 'mild retchers' who can be successfully treated with small changes to standard procedures, including:

- fast-curing impression materials
- advising patient to bend forwards in the dental chair
- use of the smallest well-fitting impression tray possible
- patient concentrating on focused breathing
- patient concentrating on a small task, such as keeping feet several inches off the chair
- relaxation and distraction
- patient practising with inert objects in the mouth.

Patients with a severe reaction may be labelled as difficult because the treatment options available are limited, despite even the best intentions and efforts of the dentist. The two major reasons responsible for disruptive gagging are somatic or psychogenic in origin. Somatic causation of gagging arises from anatomical, neurological or physiological factors, whereas psychogenic reasons for the exaggeration of the normal protective reflex stem from over-generalising from nondental stimuli, anticipatory anxiety and a visual/olfactory stimulation of the autonomic vomiting centre in the central nervous system. For gaggers with a severe response the prospect of visiting the dentist is aversive, and therefore the dentist may not come in frequent contact with these patients. The gagging response can be violent regardless of the cause. Patients report a sense of impending doom as well as a strong autonomic discharge. Features include 'extreme lacrimation, rhinorrhea, convulsive throat, abdominal, upper body and leg abduction, facial flushing, apnoea, tachycardia, escape behaviour and exhaustion' (Saunders and Cameron, 1997).

Only when the patient is in substantial dental pain or greatly aesthetically compromised will a dental visit be made possibly with a request for treatment under general anaesthetic. It is important, however, in planning treatment to assess whether the gagging response is somatic or psychogenic in origin. Treatment results will be limited if a standard mechanical approach is taken when the actual cause is anxiety-related. Assessment is facilitated by ensuring that a detailed history includes past experiences at the dentist or other medical encounters. Evidence of some past trauma in these situations may be indicative of psychological factors being implicated. A stronger anxiety response to dental procedures would be typical of the psychogenic compared to the somatic gagging patient. Personality does not appear to be a good predictor of the psychogenic patient who gags severely. Contrary to expectations, some evidence suggests that patients who are low on the personality dimension of neuroticism are more likely to suffer severe disruptive gagging, but are anxious about the dental environment.

As with other groups of patients outlined in this chapter, the importance of a good rapport between the practitioner and the patient is required. Hence, key steps in the management of the patient who gags include:

- collecting a good history of the gagging phenomena, that is – when started, association with any trauma, frequency of occurrence, trigger stimulus, method of attempted coping, worst occurrence
- inviting patients to complete a dental anxiety questionnaire – patients who gag will be more likely to score high
- if gagging appears to be psychogenic in origin then encouraging the patient to develop anxiety-reduction procedures – supervised relaxation or other self-administered techniques
- further therapeutic interventions (hypnotherapy, cognitive behavioural therapy and psychotherapy) obtainable from local health services
- topical anaesthetic over the gag trigger zone.

Are There any Solutions?

While Vignette 1 illustrates successful management of a difficult patient, dentists in general practice tend not to have the support or time necessary to enable the strengthening of the treatment alliance in such situations. Hence, at the outset it is imperative that dentists can identify patients who may be experiencing difficulties so that an appropriate course of action may be taken.

Dentists must be in a position to make an informed decision with regard to accepting or referring the patient for care. At this point, the dentist must have the necessary knowledge and communication skills to complete a patient assessment. S/he must assess the time, stress and financial costs of accepting a 'difficult' patient for continuous care. Once these assessments have been completed the dentist can make the decision to treat or to refer elsewhere for secondary-level care.

Self-Assessment

In self-assessment a decision must be made as to whether you can bear the costs (emotional, time and financial), have the appropriate communication and patient-management skills and multidisciplinary support from colleagues:

- Assessment of time and financial costs are inter-related. An assessment as to the time available for the treatment of patients with difficulties must be made. Such patients take up more time and hence add to the financial costs of the practice, with reduced throughput of patients.
- An assessment of your ability to withstand the patient's demands and complaints is needed. This may be connected to the effectiveness of your communication and patient-management skills. Communication skills are essential to forge, nurture and maintain the treatment alliance. Integrally connected with this is the awareness that the patient is displacing his or her current life difficulties onto the dentist and the practice.
- It is better to recognise limitations and possible conflicts than embarking on treatment likely to result in failure and complaints.

Assessing the New Patient

At the first interview with a new patient you should:

- Use open questions to gather all information on current life events, previous medical and dental experiences.
- Listen carefully for indicators of disappointments and complaints about other dentists. Complaints or disappointments levelled at other dentists may alert you to potential problems with the treatment you may provide.
- The use of psychological questionnaires as mentioned in Chapter 5 are useful. The Modified Dental Anxiety Scale for adults and Modified Child Dental Anxiety Scale can alert you to a child or adult who has a profound anxiety associated with dental treatment.
- Negotiate the treatment plan using frameworks such as motivational interviewing and ARMPITS (see Chapter 7). It is essential that the negotiated treatment plan is acceptable to the patient. It is at this time that the patient's

agreement must be sought. Complete records with details of the agreed treatment plan and the patient's agreement should be made.

Treat or Refer

The decision may now be taken as to whether to accept the patient into the practice or to refer to another practitioner for secondary specialist care. In some instances, whether the patient is accepted or not for treatment, the need to refer to medical colleagues will be part of the negotiated treatment plan. The requirement for close links between medical and dental colleagues provides support when treating patients with difficulties, as illustrated in the cases above.

If the decision is made to offer the patient dental treatment, the dentist must monitor his or her own responses to the patient as well as the patient's response to the care being provided. Therefore, during the course of the treatment:

* Detailed clinical notes are essential. These will include observations on the patient's response to treatment, whether complaints were made and how these complaints were handled and resolved.
* The dentist must make sure the patient understood the treatment plan, agreed to it and gave written consent to the treatment and any in-treatment amendments.
* The dentist must provide jargon-free explanations of proposed treatments. Information must be given clearly and concisely.
* The dentist must make sure the patient understands what is happening and allow him or her to voice concerns. Questions should always be answered, irrespective of how trivial and possibly irrelevant they seem.
* The dentist should assess that the patient was happy and content with the treatment outcome – for example the colour, shape of crowns, veneers and so on.

At the end of each treatment session:

* Assess whether the patient is satisfied with the care received.
* Monitor the patient's responses to treatment to ensure that the negotiated and agreed treatment has had a successful outcome.

In summary

* 'Difficult' patients are:
  - patients who have difficulties and displace them onto the dental situation

- difficult because they are demanding and complaining
- they cause disruption of the treatment alliance.

• Treatment decisions must be based on:
  - the assessment of the patient
  - an assessment of the costs of providing care
  - the dentist's ability to withstand the patient's demands and/or complaints
  - the dentist's patient-management and effective communication skills

Conclusions

The aim of this chapter was to define what was meant by the phrase 'difficult patients' and to assist the dental practitioner with decisions as to whether to accept such patients for dental care. It was suggested that patients who are difficult are patients with current life problems who may have psychological difficulties or present with oral manifestations of physical illnesses. Irrespective of the source of their problems, 'difficult patients' have the potential to disrupt the dentist-patient relationship. The ability of the dentist to understand the difficulties these patients experience can assist in providing empathetic and objective care. Therefore, using effective communication, and by discussing and negotiating proposed treatment plans with the patient, it is possible to nurture and maintain the treatment alliance and pave the way for a successful treatment outcome.

Further Reading

Chapple H, Shah S, Caress A-L, Kay EJ. Exploring dental patients' preferred roles in treatment decision-making – a novel approach. Brit Dent J 2003;194:321-327.

Kay EJ, Nuttall N. Clinical Decision-Making: An Art or Science? London: British Dental Association, 1997.

Saunders RM, Cameron J. Psychogenic gagging: Identification and treatment recommendations. Compendium 1997;18:430-440.

Chapter 7

Preventive Health Principles for Dental Practice

Aim

The aim of this chapter is to provide the reader with definitions and evidence of health education and models of health behaviour.

Outcome

At the end of this chapter the reader should know the different definitions and categories of oral health education and prevention, why oral health education is important for practice and models of health behaviour to help establish a preventive outlook and promote oral health in his/her patients.

Definitions of Health Education

The World Health Organization (WHO) has stated that the overall approach to health education should be to assist people:
• adopt and sustain healthy lifestyles
• make sensible use of health services
• make decisions both individually and collectively to improve their health status and environment.

It is within the WHO conceptual framework that dentists can promote healthier lifestyle behaviours in their patients. Why should the promotion of preventive oral health behaviours be important in everyday practice? To answer this question it is necessary to consider first the benefits from the perspective of evidence-based practice, secondly the benefits for patients and, thirdly, the benefits for dentists. Kay and Locker (1996) reviewed the dental health education literature and showed that one-to-one dental health education with patients at the chair-side helped them to adopt and sustain healthier oral lifestyles. Benefits for patients include the development of personal health skills (for example, maintenance of healthier dietary regimes), accepting responsibility for their own health (sensible use of health services) and empowerment with regard to decision-making (improvement of their own oral health status).

The promotion of oral health is associated with benefits that include shifts in policy from restoration to prevention (for example, preventive dental units, the employment of hygienists and/or oral health educators) with reductions in costs of patient care and occupational stress. Improvements in oral health of patients mirrors the development of an oral health-promoting dental practice. Under such circumstances, it is to be hoped that remuneration systems will shift to rewarding dentists for saving rather than filling teeth.

How can Practice-Based Oral Health Promotion be Achieved?

Dentists may achieve preventive health goals by using communication skills to discover the appropriate level of dental health need to allow their patients to adopt and sustain a healthier oral health lifestyle. The first step is the assessment of patient need.

Assessment of Need

Oral health education is about increasing awareness, providing health information and improving patient skills to maintain oral health. For dental health education to attain its oral health goals, the information must be tailored to the specific 'needs' of the patient.
Three different types of need exist:
- normative need - the professionally defined need. It is identified by dentists and other health professionals when they diagnose disease
- felt need – this is the lay perception of health needs, what people want and what they think needs to be done
- expressed need - the needs that people express to the dentist. These needs may be expressed in both words and actions.

Assessment of Preventive Oral Health Need

As a second step it is necessary for dentists to understand that within any population there will be healthy people, some who are at risk to disease, some who are suffering from disease and some who are getting better. Each group of patients requires a different health education input, and these various forms of prevention have been described as:
- primary prevention
- secondary prevention
- tertiary prevention.

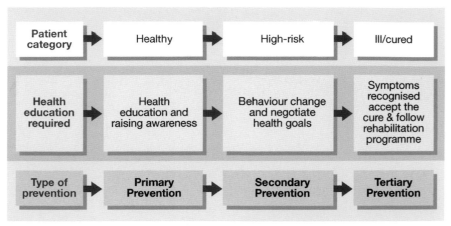

Fig 7-1 Assessment of preventive oral health need.

The type of health education will be tailored to the health and health risks of the patient. Hence, patients who are healthy may only need information to raise their awareness and to maintain their healthy status (primary prevention). Patients who are at high risk may be encouraged to take actions by the negotiation of health goals, their health behaviours and accept treatments, as may be indicated clinically (secondary prevention). Finally, patients who have been ill and recovering will need information and help to maintain their health (tertiary prevention) (Fig 7-1). In this situation a specific and tailored rehabilitation programme may be devised, with achievable health maintenance goals negotiated, agreed and set. It is necessary to decide how patients will achieve their preventive health goals. In order to help the patient do so, the dentist must be aware of the models of health behaviour that assist in the understanding of behaviour modification. This understanding will allow an appreciation of what is achievable for the patient with regard to oral health gains (for example, increase in oral health knowledge). What will be apparent in the next section is that for each category of prevention there is at least one model of health behaviour that may assist in achieving a health goal and the associated oral health gain (Fig 7-2).

Strategies for Primary Prevention: Health Behaviour Models and Health Gains

- The KAB model of health behaviour: The Knowledge, Attitude and Behaviour (KAB) model of health behaviour is based on an educational format in

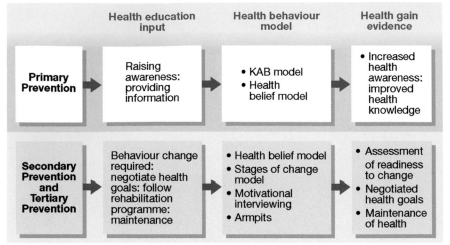

Fig 7-? Preventive oral health need, health education input, health behaviours and health gains.

which the patient is provided with health information. Previously, providing knowledge was felt to modify attitudes and enable behaviour change. This approach, however, was doomed as the provision of information was not potent enough to allow for the modification of attitudes or actions. Other reasons included the absence of acknowledging the importance of psychosocial factors. Patients from lower socio-economic groups were provided with less health advice and had shorter consultation times, which resulted in the inappropriate use of health services. The adoption of the KAB model in these circumstances resulted in an increase in health inequalities. Middle class patients were given more health education advice, were thus able to modify their attitudes and consider the adoption of new health behaviours. KAB, by not acknowledging the role of psychosocial factors in health behaviour, therefore, resulted in failure with regard to changing health actions and in increasing health inequalities.
- The health belief model and health gains: The health belief model (HBM) was conceived by Rosenstock in the 1970s. It suggested that people's health behaviour was dependent on how individuals perceived themselves with regard to the susceptibility, severity of a health condition and the benefits and costs of adopting a healthier lifestyle:
- perceived susceptibility to a health condition
- perceived severity of a health condition
- beliefs in the benefits of a health action

- beliefs concerned with the costs (time, degree of difficulty and so on) of taking a health action.

People's cues for action were based on their perceived threat of the health condition. Cues for action included media campaigns (for example, oral cancer awareness week), health education from doctor or dentist, illness of a friend or family member and/or newspaper articles.

The success of the HBM in increasing awareness has been demonstrated. It is an important tool in oral health education. Evidence for the model to promote behaviour change is, however, equivocal. Early work suggested that the HBM could not explain the prevention of periodontal disease in young women. Later research, however, has suggested that the HBM can explain preventive health behaviours in children. Difficulties with the robustness of the HBM have been linked to the fact that health care needs are traded off against other more urgent or important felt needs, including material and family needs. This meant that oral health education goals could be different for different patients as well as being different for different target groups or populations. The awareness of such influences on behaviour has led to a modification of the HBM. In this modified version, demographic (for example, socio-economic status), psychosocial (for example, dental anxiety status) and structural factors (for example, access to dental health services) are postulated as influencing variables on the adoption of preventive health actions. Therefore, in order to use the HBM to promote behaviour change, dentists must be aware of the influences of the patients':

- socio-economic background
- level of understanding/knowledge
- dental anxiety status
- attitudes to dental health
- previous dental experiences (including self-care)
- dental experiences of family and peers.

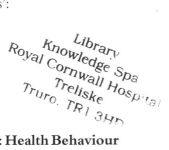

Strategies for Secondary and Tertiary Prevention: Health Behaviour Models and Health Gains

Patients' compliance with advice on oral health care is dependent on a range of demographic, psychosocial and structural factors. Bringing about lasting and effective changes in oral health behaviours is not about manipulating patients and getting them to do what dentists feel they should do. It is about exploring patients' attitudes and values in relation to their own oral health, encouraging them to identify and express their own dental health needs and empowering them to make any necessary changes in their own lives. This is the essence of the strategies that are involved in secondary and tertiary prevention. As these categories of prevention are about adopting and maintaining healthier behaviours the health behaviour models and strategies overlap and may be considered together. The health gain associated with secondary and tertiary prevention is about both behaviour change and providing health information and encouraging the adoption and maintenance of new, healthier lifestyles. These models of health behaviour acknowledge that patients have competing needs in their lives, accept that their oral health may have a low priority and that, with regard to health behaviour change, patients will be at different stages.

Stages of Change Model

The 'stages of change model' developed by Prochaska and DiClemente (1983) provides a means by which the dentist can assess the appropriate type of oral health promotion input. Intrinsic in the 'stages of change model' is the acknowledgment that competing life needs or priorities may mean that individuals may not have thought of their health or health behaviours. One of the strengths of the model is that it recognises and allows for relapsing behaviour and the redirection of action. It also requires the dentist to think beyond the KAB model of health behaviour and accept that change is an evolving process in which the dentist's role is that of facilitator.

There are five basic stages (Fig 7-3):
- The first two stages, PRE-CONTEMPLATION and CONTEMPLATION, include the period during which patients are becoming aware of the problem and the potential benefits of changing behaviour. They are not ready to change. They are also becoming aware of the alternatives available to them to help them make the necessary changes. It is wrong to assume that people already know about the alternatives open to them. This part of the process can take a long time, as it involves information-gathering and working through feelings about making changes before making any decisions.
- PREPARATION may be a lengthy process. It improves self-awareness, self-image and reduces indecisiveness. Patients must be supported, encouraged and prepared for action.
- When patients reach the ACTION AND MAINTENANCE stages they have come to realise that the benefits of changing outweighs the 'costs' to them that the change in behaviour may incur. These are not necessarily financial costs, but the fact that they have to give up what are, typically

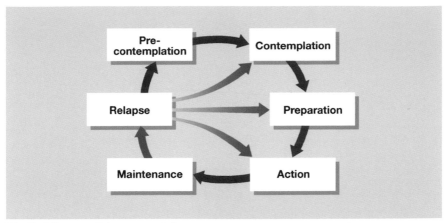

Fig 7-3 Stages of change model.

for them, enjoyable and pleasurable practices or experiences. During this part of the process the health professional is usually involved in working with patients in helping them to identify realistic goals that will encourage them to make the necessary behaviour changes.

- The RELAPSE stage occurs when (or if) maintenance strategies break down and the undesirable behaviour is resumed. This stage is quite common, particularly where the new behaviours are complex and difficult to sustain – for example, not smoking. This reinforces the need for agreeing realistic goals the patient is more likely to be able to achieve.

Application for Dental Practice
Tilliss et al (2003) have developed a four-item questionnaire to assess where patients are on the stages of change cycle. The 'Stages of Change Instrument' (SCI) defines interdental cleaning and specifically examines patients' intention, adoption and use of interdental cleaning (Fig 7-4). A key based on the patient's response is provided (Fig 7-5). This allows the dentist to place patients at a specific stage, which corresponds to their reported interdental cleaning behaviour.

The identification of the stage the patient has reached allows the dentist to tailor his/her dental health education input to the patient's oral health preventive needs. Therefore, a patient who has reached the preparation phase will need to be supported and encouraged, whereas a patient who is in contemplation will need more time. Some patients in contemplation are said to

Definition: Cleaning between your teeth is using any of the following:

• Dental floss or tape
• Toothpick
• Inter-dental sticks, inter-dental brushes
• Oral irrigator
• Other device to clean between your teeth

(NB: manual/powered toothbrushes are NOT included in this definition)

Instructions: For each of the following 4 questions, please check (√) the box corresponding to the single best answer describing your current inter-dental cleaning.

1. How frequently do you clean between your teeth?

Daily 1 ☐

3–5 times a week 2 ☐

1–2 times a week 3 ☐

Occasionally 4 ☐

Never 5 ☐

2. How long have you been cleaning between your teeth at your current frequency?

Less than 6 months 1 ☐

Between 6 months and a year 2 ☐

More than a year 3 ☐

3. In the next 30 days do you plan to clean between your teeth?

More often 1 ☐

About the same 2 ☐

Less often 3 ☐

4. In the next 6 months do you plan to clean between your teeth?

More often 1 ☐

About the same 2 ☐

Less often 3 ☐

Fig 7-4 Stages of change instrument [SCI] (Tilliss et al, 2003).

Questions Stages	**1.** How frequently do you clean between your teeth?	**2.** How long have you been cleaning between your teeth at your current frequency?	**3.** In the next 30 days do you plan to clean between your teeth?	**4.** In the next 6 months do you plan to clean between your teeth?
Maintenance	three or more times/week	six months or more		
Action	three or more times/week	< six months		
Preparation	< three times/week		More often	
Contemplation	< three times/week			More often
Precontemplation	< three times/week		About the same or less	About the same or less

Fig 7-5 Key for determining stages of change based on SCT responses.

have become 'chronic contemplators', and so it is necessary for the dental health professional to gather information and to help the patient identify and work through his/her feelings about making changes before making any decisions. If patients wish to change their behaviour it is important to understand whether or not they are ready to do so and if any barriers obstruct their way in adopting new oral health behaviours. A technique that allows the exploration of the patient's readiness to change and identification of the pros and cons of changing is motivational interviewing.

Motivational Interviewing
Behaviour change is a complex process, and in most cases is dependent on whether or not patients are ready to change. It is essential that the dentist identifies patients' competing life needs or priorities and their state of readiness to change. Doing so allows the dental health professional to provide the appropriate help and support to enable the patient to make the necessary changes.

The first step in motivational interviewing is to identify the health behaviour to be modified. In some instances this will be just one behaviour – for example, interdental cleaning - in others the patient may have a selection of behaviours to change – for example, the consumption of various cariogenic snacks and drinks. The choice of behaviour to change is the patient's.

Motivational interviewing assesses patients' readiness to change and the identification and negotiation of specific health goals. The patient's STATE OF READINESS is critical in the process of change.

At one end of the scale, it may be that patients simply require information to enable them to start to consider the possibility of change, while at the other end they may need assistance to help them identify the range of behavioural options open to them and to start to think about the benefits that change will bring. Dentists must determine the patient's state of readiness. Visual aids, such as a 'readiness rule', have been widely used. They allow an easy assessment of patients' ambivalence (UNSURE), their wish (READY) or not (NOT READY) to change.

The 'Not Ready to Change' Patient
Patients who are not ready to change must be given support and provided with health information. The time is not correct for the patient to consider adopting new oral health behaviours and the dentist must wait.

The 'Ambivalent or Unsure' Patient
The assessment of why patients feel ambivalent or unsure about changing is a central task in helping patients adopt new oral health preventive behaviours. Tilliss et al (2003) have examined patients' pros and cons for adopting interdental cleaning. The Decisional Balance Instrument (DBI) allows the dentist to understand why the patient feels unsure about changing and the barriers that obstruct behaviour modification (Fig 7-6).

Completion of the DBI identifies the attitudes against change and those for change. The awareness of issues prohibiting the forward movement in behaviour change will provide the impetus for modification in the future. This information allows the dentist to develop a tailored intervention to assist the patient on the path to readiness. For chronic contemplators this will mean having more frequent appointments to assist with, for example, techniques of interdental cleaning if they find the technique too difficult.

Here are some possible reasons why you may/not decide to clean between your teeth. For each reason, **CIRCLE** a number from 1 to 5 that shows how much each of the following reasons affects your decision to clean/not clean between your teeth 3 or more times/week.

	Does not influence me at all	Does influence hardly at all	Does influence me slightly	Does influence me quite a lot	Does influence me greatly
• To prevent bad breath	1	2	3	4	5
• To affect what others think of me	1	2	3	4	5
• To have a clean and fresh mouth	1	2	3	4	5
• To reduce visiting the dentist	1	2	3	4	5
• Difficulty in doing it	1	2	3	4	5
• To prevent gum disease	1	2	3	4	5
• The time it takes	1	2	3	4	5
• To prevent my gums bleeding	1	2	3	4	5
• To stop decay	1	2	3	4	5
• To keep my teeth	1	2	3	4	5
• Needing to look in the mirror to clean my teeth	1	2	3	4	5
• Cleaning between my teeth makes my gums bleed	1	2	3	4	5
• My fingers don't fit into my mouth	1	2	3	4	5
• The desire for whiter teeth	1	2	3	4	5
• My mouth looks nicer	1	2	3	4	5
• My family's opinions about my mouth are important to me	1	2	3	4	5
• Difficulty in remembering to do it	1	2	3	4	5
• Cleaning between my teeth is messy	1	2	3	4	5
• So I can chew my food	1	2	3	4	5
• Pride in commitment to do it	1	2	3	4	5
• To improve/maintain my self-confidence	1	2	3	4	5
• It keeps others out of the bathroom	1	2	3	4	5
• Its frustrating cleaning between my teeth	1	2	3	4	5
• It hurts my gums	1	2	3	4	5
• It saves me money on dental care	1	2	3	4	5
• Because I like my teeth	1	2	3	4	5
• It makes dental visits less worrying	1	2	3	4	5

Fig 7-6 Decisional balance instrument [DCI] (Tilliss et al, 2003).

The 'Ready to Change' Patient

Dentists must help 'ready to change' patients identify the health behaviours they wish to change. The choice of the behaviour to be changed belongs with the patient. The dentist's role is to point out potential areas of behaviour modification. When the choice has been made, the patient has ownership of the decision. The next steps in the negotiation procedure will promote patient empowerment. With success in the modification and maintenance of one behaviour, the patient will be empowered to change the next one on the list, until all health goals and their associated health gains have been achieved. Improvements in self-esteem and life-skills have been reported to accompany improved oral health status.

When the dental health professional has identified the patient who wishes to change and the specific health behaviour to be modified then the time has come to NEGOTIATE THE BEHAVIOUR CHANGE. Health goals are an important aspect when negotiating behaviour change. They are said to be the 'staging posts' on the way to sustained behaviour change. Negotiating behaviour change falls somewhere between advice-giving and counselling. When the patient's and dentist's agendas are totally different, difficulties will be encountered. Therefore, the patient must be directly involved in identifying the behaviours to be modified and in setting his/her own health goals.

Models for Negotiating Health Goals: The 'ARMPITS' Strategy

- ARMPITS, developed from assertiveness training programmes, is a tool to negotiate acceptable and achievable health goals by the patient and dentist. Therefore, if health goals are to be achieved they must be Appropriate, Realistic, Measurable, Positive, Important, Time-related, Specific and Supported.
- The negotiated health goals are agreed within a time frame that is specific, important, acceptable and realistic for the patient and is measurable by both the patient and dentist. Within the negotiation, the dentist is positive and provides support for the emerging new behaviour. In this way ARMPITS becomes an integral part of motivational interviewing and the preparation, action and maintenance phase of the stages of change model.
- Adopting more dynamic models of health behaviour, in contrast to more linear models of health education, allows an appreciation of the patients' difficulties in changing and sustaining behaviour modification. The stages-of-change model and motivational interviewing acknowledge that behaviour change is difficult. The attainment of increased oral health

knowledge or transient improvements in oral health actions are positive health gains. With time, newly adopted oral health behaviours will be sustained and patients will have developed personal health skills, be able to use health services appropriately, and be empowered with regard to making informed choices about their oral health status.

Guidelines to Best Practice when Negotiating Behaviour Change

(1) Dental health professionals must avoid making assumptions about the patient. These assumptions include:
* that the patient ought to change, is ready to change and is either motivated to change or not
* dental health is a motivating factor
* the consultation has failed if there is no agreement to change
* now is the right time for the patient to consider change
* a tough/frightening approach is always best
* 'I'm the expert - my advice must be followed'.

(2) Principles of good practice in negotiating behaviour change include:
* respect for patients' autonomy and their choices
* readiness to change is essential and is taken into account
* patient ambivalence to change is common and reasons need to be explored and understood
* target/goals should be identified by the patient
* the expert provides information and support
* the patient is the active decision-maker.

Conclusions

The aim of this chapter was to provide definitions and evidence as to why dental health professionals should consider adopting a preventive philosophy in their everyday clinical practice. Evidence was presented as to the benefits to the patient and the practice. A series of steps were suggested, ranging from an understanding of the concept of need and prevention to a framework that incorporated various models of health behaviour. These assist in providing appropriate oral health education input and to understand the difficulties people have in changing their behaviours. Putting these concepts and ideas into practice allows the development and establishment of preventive health principles in oral health care.

Further Reading

Kay EJ, Locker D. Is dental health education effective? A systematic review of current evidence. Community Dent Oral Epidemiol 1996;24:231-235.

Prochaska JO, Diclemente CC. Stages and processes of self-change of smoking: toward an integrative model of change. Journal of Consulting and Clinical Psychology 1983;5:390-395.

Tilliss TSI, Stach DJ, Cross-Poline GN et al. The Transtheoretical Model applied to an oral self-care behavioral change: development and testing of instruments for stages of change and decisional balance. Journal of Dental Hygiene 2003;77:16-26.

Table 8-1 **Daily dosage of fluoride dietary supplements**

Daily dosage schedule for area with less than 0.3ppm fluoride in the water supply:	
6 months to 3 years:	0.25mg F (0.5mg NaF)
3 years up to 6 years:	0.5mg F (1.1mg NaF)
Over 6 years of age:	1.0mg F (2.2mg NaF)

Table 8-2 **Concentrations of fluoride toothpastes**

Category of toothpaste	Concentration (ppm F)	Target group
Low concentration pastes	<600ppm F	Low caries risk children under the age of seven, particularly if living in a water fluoridated area
Higher concentration pastes	1000–1450ppm F	High caries risk children under the age of seven (parents must use only a small pea-size amount of toothpaste)
	1450ppm F	Children over the age of seven or older
Highest concentration pastes	2800ppm F	High caries risk adults and older people

sised, together with the need for parents to supervise brushing and to encourage the children to spit the toothpaste out rather than rinsing with water.

4. Fluorsis – information is provided with regard to the relationship between excessive ingestion of fluoride during enamel formation and fluorsis.

Dietary control:

1. Sugars and dental caries – scientific evidence is provided to demonstrate the relationship between dental caries and the frequent ingestion of cariogenic sugars. Cariogenic sugars are defined as 'non-milk extrinsic sugars'. These include sucrose, glucose, fructose, maltose, dextrose, invert sugar, hydrolysed starch and so on. They are contained in foods containing added sugars at the time of manufacture, table sugar, fruit juices, pulps, purée, honey and so on.
2. Non-cariogenic sweeteners are listed and include – for example, mannitol, sorbitol, xylitol and so on. Xylitol, in particular, is important in the reduction of dental caries as small dietary additions lead to impressive reductions in caries incidence.
3. Frequency of sugar intake is highlighted, together with the use of sugar-free medicines.

Plaque control:

1. Plaque control and dental disease - the relationship between plaque, dental caries and periodontal disease is unravelled. The document endorses the removal of plaque in the prevention of periodontal disease but cautions against plaque removal in the prevention of dental caries: 'The results have been inconclusive and have failed to demonstrate a clear association between regular and efficient toothbrushing and a low caries experience'.
2. The value of toothbrushing in the prevention of dental caries is as a vehicle for fluoride toothpaste.
3. Plaque removal – detailed information is given on the type of toothbrush, interdental cleaning and techniques to be used in plaque removal for children and adults.
4. Mouthwashes or chemical plaque suppressants are described and discussed, with evidence being provided with regard to their efficacy and use.

Erosion:

1. Dietary factors are highlighted as being primary in the causation of dental erosion. If gastric regurgitation is suspected, referral to a medical practitioner is essential.
2. Erosion may be prevented by reducing the intake of erosive drinks and foods. Children, adolescents and young adults should be targeted and encouraged to drink beverages through a straw.
3. Resistance to erosion can be increased by the use of topical fluorides - for example, fluoride toothpaste and/or mouthwashes - or by professional application of fluoride varnishes and gels.

4. Brushing to be avoided for one hour after the 'acidic episode'.

Advice for denture wearers:
1. Routine care of dentures: the document stresses that the routine care of dentures should include cleaning after meals and before sleeping. It endorses the use of brushes and liquid soap to clean dentures before soaking in hypochlorite solutions. The remaining natural teeth should be cleaned with a suitable toothbrush and fluoride toothpaste.
2. Dental attendance: complete-denture wearers should attend for oral examination on a yearly basis.

Oral cancer:
1. Epidemiological information is provided with regard to prevalence and incidence of oral cancer.
2. Emphasis is placed upon the importance of the frequency of tobacco and alcohol consumption as primary risk factors in oral cancer.
3. The need for early diagnosis is endorsed.
4. Smoking cessation and moderation of alcohol consumption recommended.

Preventing Dental Diseases in Primary Dental Care

In general dentists adopt a 'high-risk' approach to prevention. Adult and child patients who are perceived to be at risk of oral disease tend to be identified and provided with appropriate preventive intervention. Rather than being proactive and raising awareness in patients to prevent dental caries, periodontal disease (say, primary prevention), dentists tend to be reactive to the disease process and provide interventions which are secondary (for example, promoting interdental cleaning) or tertiary (for example, placing fissure sealants). The means by which dentists assess their patients' treatment needs (normative need) will not be described here, but it is apparent that an integral part of promoting oral health is the assessment of the patient's oral health status.

Little information is available on the primary preventive practices of general dental practitioners. Dental health education in the form of awareness-raising and information provision tends to take place in other settings. Research concerned with active (for example, tooth-brushing skills) and passive (for example, fissure sealants) secondary and tertiary preventive care is, however, available. It is here that concerns are raised with regard to dentists' use of evidence-based research and established policy in their practice. In general, the literature suggests that dentists in Europe tend to pro-

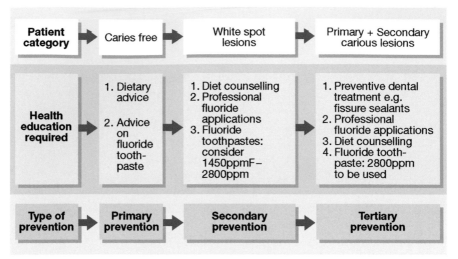

Fig 8-1 Prevention of dental caries in dental practice.

vide oral hygiene instruction, use fluorides and dietary advice as preventive strategies for children who they consider to be at high-risk of caries (Fig 8-1).

More recent work suggests, however, that high-risk children from lower socio-economic groups are more likely to be found to receive only oral hygiene instruction, whereas those from middle or high socio-economic groups are provided with professionally applied topical fluorides. Nevertheless, as caries risk increases children are more likely to receive dietary advice, fluoride supplements and professionally applied fluoride treatments. Furthermore, it seems that dentists are unsure of the guidelines with regard to fluoride toothpaste use if children are living in an area of water fluoridation. The question remains: how can evidence-based research and guidelines be incorporated into everyday clinical practice? It seems that guidelines and evidence–based research are not necessarily the major influences upon the preventive interventions made by dentists in practice. Does it all boil down to fees, and if dentists were suitably remunerated would it enable them to adopt a preventive approach? Nevertheless, dentists need accessible information and evidence-based recommendations to promote prevention and team work.

Preventing Dental Caries

- Dental caries and dietary counselling: Watt and McGlone (2003) provide the evidence on 'dietary interventions' for dental practice. They state that the difficulties that dentists experience are related to problems in translating oral health knowledge into action. Watt and McGlone (2003) suggest a series of practical steps, including identifying the high-risk patient, dietary history, setting goals, developing an action plan, monitoring and review and referring if necessary (see Chapter 7). Most importantly, they point to the inclusion of all of the members of the dental team and fostering a team approach. The requirement for dentists to acknowledge the role of hygienists, therapists and oral health educators in providing dietary counselling for the child and adult high-risk patient is emphasised.
- Dental caries and fluoride toothpaste: Dentists should encourage twice-daily toothbrushing with a fluoride toothpaste. Davies at al (2003) provide clear, evidence-based guidelines on the use of fluoride toothpaste in the prevention of dental caries. They propose that patients must be encouraged to brush their teeth twice a day with fluoride toothpaste and that the concentration of fluoride toothpaste be determined by the age and caries risk of the patient.

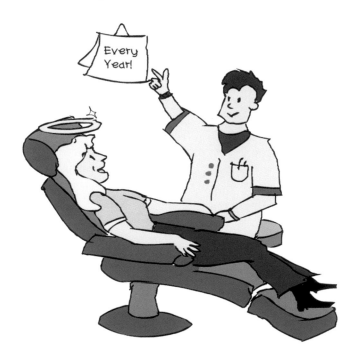

- Parents should be told to brush their children's teeth as soon as the first deciduous teeth erupt. Children's toothbrushing should be supervised (with a pea-size amount of toothpaste used). The use of high-concentration fluoride toothpastes for older people, perceived to be at risk from dental caries is recommended. Mouth-rinsing with water should be discouraged. Teeth should be brushed using a fluoride toothpaste on going to bed and at one other time of the day. In addition, older patients with moderate to high risk of dental caries should be encouraged to rinse daily with fluoride mouthwash. The need for teamwork and the role of hygienists is important in the promotion of regular fluoride toothpaste use.
- Dental caries and professionally applied fluorides: Professionally applied fluorides are indicated for patients with a high risk of dental caries on smooth surfaces and exposed root surfaces, who have a reduced salivary flow, are receiving orthodontic treatment and for whom fissure sealants are unsuitable. The types of topical fluoride include fluoride varnishes (effective in high-caries-risk children and older people) and fluoride gels (effective in high-caries-risk children). In their paper Hawkins et al (2003) provide detailed information on the assessment of the high-risk patient.
- Dental caries and fissure sealants: Locker et al (2003) provide guidelines for the use of fissure sealants as well as the cost-effectiveness of this preventive intervention. They describe the effectiveness of fissure sealants and suggest that autopolymerising (chemical-cure) sealants have the longest retention rates. Detailed information is given with regard to the type of child requiring fissure sealants, when sealants should be placed, which surfaces should be sealed and the techniques involved.

Preventing Periodontal Disease

- Plaque removal and periodontal disease: Davies et al (2003) state that dentists should aim to provide dental health education and tooth-brushing skills to enable their patients 'to maintain a level of plaque control which ensures that the rate of tissue destruction is reduced sufficiently to ensure . . . a comfortable and functional dentition'.

In order to achieve this aim it is recommended that patients are advised to brush their teeth twice daily, to brush their teeth in a systematic manner to ensure plaque removal, to use a toothbrush with a small head, soft, long and short round-ended filaments and a comfortable handle. The use of powered toothbrushes is mentioned. Those unable to maintain an effective level of plaque control should be advised to use a powered toothbrush. It is suggested that toothpastes containing triclosan and zinc citrate should be recommended to patients unable to control their plaque levels, as they assist in improving plaque control.

• Mouthwashes and periodontal disease: The adjunct use of antimicrobial mouthwashes can provide benefits to patients who are unable to maintain adequate levels of plaque control through tooth brushing alone. Dentists should recommend products that have proven clinical effectiveness.

Promoting Dental Attendance

When promoting access to care, dentists need to consider practice policy with regard to the types of dental health personnel employed, the geographic location of the practice, continuing professional development and patients' service needs, such as evening or Saturday surgeries. Awareness that the patient's psychological profile (for example, dental anxiety status) and social factors (socio-economic status) are likely to influence dental attendance can assist the practice in reducing barriers and promoting accessibility. Practical suggestions for encouraging dental registration and dental attendance have included:

• Practice open days to allow patients to view the practice facilities, together with information leaflets and postcards providing practice details and services, have been shown to be important in improving access to care.
• Practice websites: Excellent examples of practice websites are to be found on http://www.derweb.co.uk/twork/news.html. The websites provide details on the practice, its position (in some instances with maps), treatment and facilities, as well as introducing the members of the dental team. Dental health information is given, together with assurances about dental anxiety and sedation services.
• Multidisciplinary working: Health visitors working with mothers and liaising closely with dentists can advise and recommend practices in areas close to the family home. Dentists taking part in such initiatives have been impressed by the increase in registration of preschool children.

Oral Cancer, Opportunistic Screening and Smoking Cessation

Oral cancer is the sixth most common cancer worldwide. It has devastating consequences for patients, with an overall survival rate of 50%, and deleterious effects on general and health-related quality of life. Treatment improvements are assessed by enhancement to life quality as opposed to increased survival-years. This is because it has been difficult to demonstrate major advances in survival. Hence, the major thrust to reducing death rates for oral cancer relies on prevention of the disease. Patients delaying investigation for suspected lesions place themselves at greater risk, as more severe disease strengthens the likelihood of increased mortality. Early identification of cancerous or pre-cancerous lesions through population screening has been recognised as uneconomic. However, efforts should be directed to increase the accessibility for opportunistic screening – the systematic checking of the mouths of all patients attending for dental care. This approach, however, limits the availability of screening, as it is restricted to those who visit the dentist.

People over the age of 40, smokers and alcoholics have been suggested as target groups to receive educational interventions. Knowledge of oral cancer in these individuals is low, in particular a lack of awareness about warning signs and symptoms.

The dissemination of carefully designed patient information leaflets has resulted in improving knowledge and willingness to have a screen. Contrary to expectations, informing patients about oral cancer in this way reduces rather than increases anxiety. Interestingly, those who benefit the most from these information campaigns are those at higher risk, in particular, smokers.

Oral Cancer: Opportunistic Screening
The practitioner and the dental team need a joint approach to assessing the patient's oral health, especially for the presence of cancerous lesions. Examples of a practice approach would be:
1. The practice literature to new patients include information on the screening procedures
2. All patients arriving for an oral health check are given a short explanation of the aims of the procedure. This will detail both the assessment of untreated caries, periodontal disease, malocclusion viral and bacterial infections and other lesions (that are rare), which can usually and typically be treated successfully if identified early
3. A policy, drawn up by the practice team, to explain to practice personnel their responsibilities when a patient is identified to have a possible malignant lesion. The policy would give guidelines to new associates, hygienists, receptionists and nursing staff. For example, receptionists should be alerted if a patient has been sent to the local teaching hospital for biopsy, so that if the patient telephones the practice s/he is given opportunity to speak to the dentist who referred her/him for the specialist opinion. In order to achieve this goal the receptionist should be asked to mark the patient's chart or, if a computer system is used, to 'flag' the patient's record.

Oral Cancer: Dealing with a Positive Diagnosis

Having the practice tuned in to a policy of conducting routine checks for suspicious lesions should also have a section outlining how to manage a patient when s/he is positively identified as suffering from oral cancer. In Chapter 3 the breaking of bad news was described as a process that had some recommendations for good practice. The overall message was that practitioners presented themselves as genuinely concerned and caring. Examples of this approach in the care of the patient with oral cancer would be for the dental practitioner to contact and invite the patient to the practice to discuss any questions while waiting for the specialist clinic appointment. The dentist may ask the patient to let the practice know of the outcome of the clinic appointment and also to share any concerns during the waiting period prior to the result of a biopsy or other tests that may have been conducted.

Oral Cancer: Intervention for Smoking Cessation

Some brief interventions that have been used successfully in primary dental care use the four 'A's and two 'R's (Fig 8-2).

In practical terms the dentist must:
ASK patients about their smoking habits:
- Are you a smoker?
- How many cigarettes do you smoke?

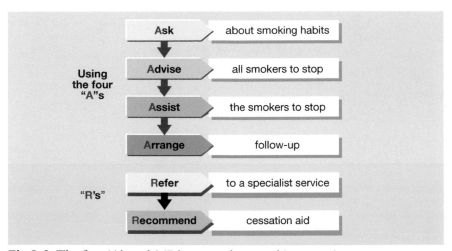

Fig 8-2 The four 'A's and 2 'R's approach to smoking cessation.

- When you wake up, when do you have your first cigarette?
- Have you ever tried to stop smoking?
- Would you like to try to stop now?'

ADVISE all smokers on the value of stopping smoking:
The information given should be specific, understandable and personal to each patient. Health education should include the benefits of quitting, such as fresher breath, healthier skin, less staining on teeth and healthier gums, feeling better, having more energy, reduced risk from cancers and heart disease, better healing, breaking the dependency on nicotine and more disposable income.

ASSIST those smokers who want to stop with appropriate support:
The assessment of the smoker's readiness to stop can be made using the readiness rule as described in Chapter 7. For those who are ready to try to change their smoking habits dentists can assist by providing details on nicotine replacement therapy, bupropion (Zyban), telephone support lines and health education materials on quitting. The support of the hygienist is essential as s/he can negotiate a quitting date with the patient, review previous quitting attempts, stress the importance of the support of family and friends and provide in-depth health education as well as negotiating health goals.

ARRANGE monitoring, follow-up and referral if appropriate:
The dentist can arrange for patients to be referred to specialist smoking cessation services (such as health promotion agencies and cancer charities). The dentist, working with the hygienist, can arrange to monitor the patient's progress at regular intervals.

Conclusions

The aim of this chapter was to provide the dentist with evidenced-based policy and recommendations with regard to providing preventive interventions in primary dental care. The policy document *The Scientific Basis of Oral Health Education* was summarised and recommendations for practice suggested. Practical suggestions have been made together with the emphasis for a team approach in the prevention oral diseases in everyday clinical practice.

Further Reading

The Scientific Basis of Dental Health Education: A Policy Document (revised 4th Edition):
* www.dpb.nhs.uk/archives/other/sci_basis_dental_health1.pdf
* www.dpb.nhs.uk/archives/other/sci_basis_dental_health2.pdf

Kay E. A Guide to Prevention in Dentistry (including The Scientific Basis of Oral Health Education) London: BDJ Books, 2004.

For general practice website designs:
* www.derweb.co.uk/twork/news.html

Smoking cessation websites and helplines:
* Restorative Dentistry Oncology, www.rdoc.org.uk
* Faculty of Dental Surgery, Royal College of Surgeons of England. Clinical Guidelines: the management of oncology patients – www.rcseng.ac.uk/dental/fds/clinical_guidelines

Quitline:
+44 (0) 800 00 2200

NHS Smoking Helpline:
+44 (0) 800 169 0169

Watt RG, Daly B. Prevention. Part 1: Smoking cessation advice within the general dental practice. Brit Dent J 2003;194:665–668.

Watt RG, McGlone S. Prevention. Part 2: Dietary advice in the dental surgery. Brit Dent J 2003;195:27–31.

Davies RM, Davis GM, Ellwood RP. Prevention Part 4: Toothbrushing: What advice should be given to patients? Brit Dent J 2003;195:135–141.

Hawkins R, Locker D, Noble J. Prevention. Part 7: Professionally applied topical fluorides for caries prevention. Brit Dent J 2003;195:313–317.

Locker D, Jokovic A. Prevention. Part 8: The use of pit and fissure sealants in preventing caries in permanent dentition of children. Brit Dent J 2003;195:375–378.

Chapter 9
Communication, Stress and Improved Patient Care

Aim

To outline the basis of self-care for dental health professionals to enable them to function optimally and deliver high-quality oral health care provision.

Outcome

After reading this chapter readers should better understand what factors, external and internal to their workplace, influence their psychological well-being and be able to apply recommended ways of assessing and coping with occupational pressures, in the short and long term. In addition, on a broader level, readers should understand the benefits of introducing applied psychological principles to maintain a satisfactory level of physical health and mental well-being and, in turn, sustain the standard of care for their patients. Occupational psychologists, such as Cary Cooper, have studied the relationship between stress, ill health and changes in clinical dental practice. The widespread belief that dentistry is the most stressful of all health professions is not without some foundation, although there is considerable variation among individuals and practices. Dentists are, for instance, more likely to have problems with dependency on alcohol and drugs, suffer from coronary heart disease, commit suicide and be divorced compared with members of the general population. Recent evidence suggests that the claim that dentists score less favourably on these health-related indices is unconvincing when compared to other professional groups, including accountants and lawyers.

Stress has a multifaceted definition – 'results from an imbalance between the demands made of individuals and their perceived ability to cope'. Stress can be considered as an affective response to significant life events, such as a road traffic accident, bereavement or divorce. Any of these events can trigger a stress reaction. Stress can also be construed as a physical response with the well-known physiological reactions of flight or fight. The recognition of the potential sources of occupational stress enables practitioners to possess the means to reduce stress and thereby prevent the condition of burnout.

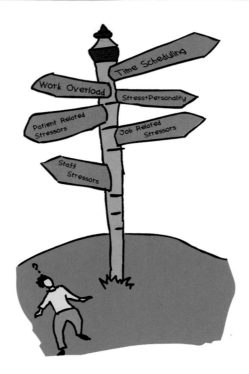

Sources of Occupational Dental Stress

Wilson's study highlighted the stressors for over 1,000 general dental practitioners in England and Wales, the large majority of whom were working in NHS practices. Respondents indicated the degree of pressure from over 30 occupational stressors within dental practice. The use of identical questions enabled comparison with an earlier study by Cooper and his research team. Results are summarised in Table 9-1.

Wilson's study showed that workload and time pressures were the most frequently rated pressures. Associated with these were stressors summarising income-related issues (for instance, managing financial demands, balancing the accounts and so on) and difficult patients. These stressors can be grouped into five areas (see Table 9-2). The following sections describe some of the factors in more detail under each heading.

Table 9-1 **Top ten stressors for practitioners in England and Wales** (Wilson et al 1998)

Stressor	Percent considerably stressed or more	Rank order	Rank order UK comparison study (1986)*
Running behind schedule	62	1	3
Working constraints set by the NHS	58	2	-
Coping with difficult or uncooperative patients	57	3	2
Working quickly to see as many patients as possible	51	4	-
Working under constant time pressures	51	5	4
Patient having a medical emergency in surgery	51	6	1
Seeing more patients than you want to for income reasons	50	7	-

*   study by Cooper et al British Dental Journal 1987; 184:499-502

Table 9-2 **Mean score for each group of stressors**

Stressor group	Mean score
Time-related	3.49
Income-related	3.24
Patient-related	3.23
Job-related	2.64
Staff/technical-related	2.51

Workload

Excessive workload has been described as simply having too much work to do or, from a qualitative perspective, work being too difficult for the individual. Quantitatively, dental occupational stress can be experienced through the pressure of time in treating patients. The NHS system of payment - fee per item, or piecework - significantly increases dentists' work overload as the tendency to see more patients and undertake more procedures to cover practice overheads is high. Qualitatively, work overload is associated with dentists having to compromise their working practices from an ideal that they learnt in dental school to what can be delivered under the constraints of a system of remuneration. The longer-term outcome is poor assessment of the patient's previous dental experiences, dental anxiety status, expressed or felt needs. This may eventually lead to difficulties with patients. Dentists, because of their own life experiences and personalities, will either be able or not to cope with criticisms of their professional integrity. Dentists who are anxious will react with hostility to patients with high dental anxiety status. Dentists whose work is criticised by patients will react with disappointment and anger. Such experiences are perceived as being stressful by both dentist and patient.

Work underload is associated with boring and repetitive work observed in occupations such as dentistry. Dentists who are not sufficiently challenged intellectually by their work can experience occupational stress. Paradoxically, work underload can therefore be a stressor.

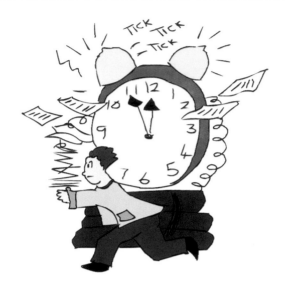

Time-Scheduling

Dentists seek to become more efficient and consider fitting more patients into their diaries. Among recently qualified dentists the competition for dental patients is strong. The new dentist in general practice must cover the costs of setting up and running a dental practice and so must encourage a full appointment book. An appointment missed, let alone time off due to sickness or other reason, will in effect be lost income. Cooper et al (1987) demonstrated that 'running behind schedule' and 'constant time pressures' ranked third and fourth, respectively, out of over 30 potential stressors by dentists in general dental practice. Wilson et al (1998) showed that time-related stressors were the most highly rated. Sixty-two percent reported that 'running behind schedule' was 'considerably stressful'.

Job-Related Stressors

In general, being knowledgeable about new technologies, attending meetings, reading journals and keeping up with new materials and clinical techniques have all been recognised as vital tasks for dentists. Continuing professional development has become mandatory in many countries. There may be wide variation in response to these demands. Attendance at meetings can provide a necessary break from routine and a time to gain support from peers in general discussion periods. Some dentists may regard such activities as interrupting the business of their practice.

Changes in work regimes (fee for item to insurance schemes,) together with new technologies, are additional stressors for the dentist. Further examples of changes to working practices that are increasing demands are time taken up with completing paperwork, being on call, continuous care and capitation, and longer working hours.

Sources of dental occupational stress in the surgery environment may include:
- time taken for materials to set and radiographs to develop
- the noise from both high and low-speed handpieces
- equipment that fails to operate optimally
- constant attention to small detail
- manual dexterity and close working
- procedures and devices not working properly
- the persistent glare of the operating lights
- the smells of dental materials.

Beyond the immediate environment of the dental chair, the design and layout of the surgery and other factors, such as the ventilation or air conditioning system, can all either reduce or exacerbate stress. Communication networks will be influenced by the layout and design of the dental surgery, waiting room and staff areas. The nature of dental treatment with its concentration on fine detail and close work can cause eyestrain and headaches. The changes in levels and frequency of noise more than a constant pitch can act as an irritant. Concerns about close contact with certain materials such as mercury, nitrous oxide, anaesthetic gases and more importantly fears of contamination infection with diseases such as HIV, hepatitis and tuberculosis may all contribute to staff anxiety in the dental environment.

Patient-Related Stressors

Cooper et al (1987) stated that 'When someone is constantly aware of potential danger, s/he is prepared to react immediately. The individual is in a constant state of arousal'. Dentists are in a constant state of arousal, never being sure what the next appointment will bring - the phobic patient, adverse reactions to antibiotic treatment and so on. For some, this can be a means to retain an interest in their job, while others may regard this as a burden. Moreover, having close working contact with patients means that dentists may inhale particles of dental debris, bacterial aerosols and microbial products. Concerns about effective cross-infection control are also potential causes for stress and anxieties.

Staff/Technical-Related Stressors

Stress in the workplace can arise due to difficulties in defining the individual's working role, resulting in ambiguity, conflict and questions over the degree of responsibility for others.

Role ambiguity arises as a result of unrealistic expectations of the scope and extent of the work. For dentists this happens when they change status from associate to partner, or when a dental nurse becomes the practice manager. These individuals will experience role ambiguity since they will have to take on the role of 'boss' while still working with people who have been colleagues and friends.

Role conflict is a consequence of conflicting demands associated with work. Specifically for dentists this means 'inter-role conflict' and 'role overload'. Dentists have various roles within the dental practice, including administrator, employer, carer and colleague. Moreover, dentists will be responsible for the practice premises, the dental equipment and materials, the finances, salaries, for the staff members, themselves and the patients. Since dentists are required to play all these different parts during any one working day, such role diversity often results in occupational stress.

Closely associated with role diversity are the relationships dentists experience at work. Working relationships can be both potential sources of occupational stress or act as buffers. These working relationships exist at various levels, ranging from the employer to colleague to friend and supporter. Effective management and good communication will enhance the quality of these relationships. Due to the nature of dental care dentists work with one dental nurse. When this is a good working relationship the dental nurse preempts the dentist's needs during the provision of treatment. The receptionist also assists the dentist with appropriate appointment times for patients. Poor communication between the members of the dental team can result in unaired staff grievances and inefficient working practices. These will inevitably increase occupational stress.

Stress and Personality

No two people react to an event in exactly the same way. There is substantial variation in the way individuals perceive specific stressors. Dentists who enjoy variety in their work and seek challenge will rate new practice developments positively, whereas other dentists will find changes

Table 9-3 **Features of type A and type B personalities**

Type A people tend to be	Type B people tend to be
hard-driving	ambitious
extremely competitive	successful
high-achieving	no time urgency
aggressive, hasty, impatient	relaxed, patient, calm
chronically hassled	work without agitation
high expectations of themselves and others	'relax without guilt'

difficult to cope with. Personality differences between individuals can help to explain this variation. In the early 1960s Friedman and Rosenman developed a personality profile for the susceptibility to coronary heart disease. They identified two main personality types, which they described as type A and type B (Table 9-3).

People experience relative degrees of type A and type B behaviours. In other words, a continuum exists between type A at one end and type B at the other. Most people lie somewhere along this line. Awareness of your type A personality profile and of those who work with you may help to understand the likely stress response to changes around you and among members of the practice.

Responses to Stress

- A certain amount of everyday stress is compatible with good health and is necessary for coping with the challenges of everyday life. Problems start to occur when the stress response is inappropriate to the size of the challenge. As the optimum level of stress is exceeded, performance rapidly deteriorates.

Table 9-4 **Signs of burnout**

Physical signs	Emotional signs
sleeplessness, exhaustion	irritable, outbursts of anger
tension headaches	tearful
breathlessness	avoid commitment to care
skin complaints	cynicism
aches and pains	decrease in empathy
gastrointestinal disturbances	poor job satisfaction

* There are three phases of response to everyday stress, known as the general adaptation syndrome. These phases are:
  - initial alarm reaction - associated with the adrenaline kick of the flight or fight reaction
  - resistance - the mind and body cope with the stress in a sustained way. If the stress is too intense and lasts for too long the body's adaptive reserves become depleted, stress becomes distress and illness is likely.
  - exhaustion is routinely seen in health professionals with 'burn-out'.

What is Burnout?

Burnout has been described by Cherniss as 'a disease of overcommitment' associated with 'withdrawal from work in response to excessive stress or dissatisfaction'. It is an example of an inappropriate stress response to the challenge of work and is associated with poor work performance and illness. It has been proposed that burnout occurs in all health professionals at some time during their professional lives. Burnout results in higher rates of employee turn-over and absenteeism as well as decreased effectiveness and lowered morale. There are a number of physical and emotional signs (see Table 9-4).

Practitioners can assess their own level of burnout by accessing one of the websites below. In the Netherlands the development of a dental website to assess and provide sensitive feedback to dentists on possible burnout levels is at an advanced stage. Some more general measures are available, such as the Maslach Burnout Inventory (MBI), and are used in surveys, principally of those who work closely in the caring professions. The data collected are compared to norms compiled for various countries (for example, USA, UK and the Netherlands). Substantial knowledge has been gained of the MBI, which produces a helpful breakdown of the concept of burnout into three overlapping dimensions:

1. emotional exhaustion - a state of complete fatigue associated with exposure to patient distress
2. depersonalisation - a sense of being remote and cut off from the patient's experience
3. lack of personal achievement - practitioners feel their anticipated goals are not realisable.

According to Maslach, the individuals have to score in the top one third of each of the three components to be classified as suffering burnout. Estimates of the extent of burnout in dentists vary according to the measure adopted and the method of setting the upper tertile (population norm or using the survey sample to determine the cut-off levels). Studies in the Netherlands, Scandinavia and the UK show that approximately 10–15% of dentists satisfy the criteria of burnout. Evidence from the Netherlands shows that short-term intervention (minimal counselling and group discussion) can prevent burnout. It has also been argued that depersonalisation, one of the elements of burnout, may be an effective coping mechanism for a proportion of dentists, but unfortunately this method of managing the patient contact is detrimental to the therapeutic alliance mentioned previously and may be counter-productive to the dentist in the long term.

Coping with Occupational Stress and Burnout

Features of burnout, such as depersonalisation, can be a temporary method of coping. More serious is when dentists are unaware that they are adopting this strategy. This is an example of the tendency of all health professionals to deny occupational stress. Awareness-raising is therefore important. Within the busy general dental practice it is beneficial if dentists are able to assess efficiently the degree of occupational stress being experienced by their staff and themselves. This prevents repeated stressful experiences that can

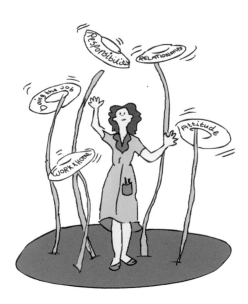

result in burnout and mental health problems. The first step in controlling occupational stress is recognising the demands made on you by patients and staff, an assessment of those demands, the means of coping with the demands and the outcomes of the coping strategies used.

These may include:
- assessing and evaluating the environmental demands made on you at any one time during the working day - such as workload, job performance, being responsible for patients, staff and family
- assessing the emotional outcomes of these demands – do you perceive them as being threatening, irrelevant, challenging, hostile, friendly and enhancing self-esteem?
- assessing the type of controlling/coping methods you use to deal with the demands made on you - the effects of these coping strategies both in the short term and long term and the outcomes and influences they have upon your occupational stress, working practices and physical health.

There are various behavioural strategies that can be used as means of coping with occupational stress. The main strategies that may be used are relaxation, assertiveness and problem-solving.

Associated with problem-solving is the recognition of demands made on the team through work and our personal habitual ways of coping. For the principal this could include:

- calling a practice meeting to discuss the issue of stress in the workplace
- performing a stress 'audit' through group discussion or completion of standardised questionnaires
- identifying, with other members of your dental team, these sources of stress
- setting out a number of realistic goals with a method of ascertaining whether the goal is being met.

For example, the team may identify that managing emergency patients is a cause of great pressure within the practice because of misunderstandings among the staff of the usual procedure that has been employed in the past. The team may consider that a policy needs to be written and a date set for piloting and eventual implementation.

The associate, for example, may find working 'after hours' difficult to honour because of family commitments. S/he could explore with the principal the possibility of offering longer working hours on set nights only.

Recognition of Danger Signs: Alcohol and Drug Abuse

There are recommendations for healthy drinking (21 units for men and 14 units for women - one unit is a glass of wine or half a pint of beer). Where individuals are consuming above these levels on a regular and long-term basis they should examine closely what factors might be causing consistent high levels of consumption. Danger signals for excessive alcohol consumption include sweats, tremors, phases of memory loss and poor concentration, rapid mood swings, depression and angry outbursts. Other work colleagues may be first to notice these changes and may assist by suggesting independent and confidential help. In the UK such help may be obtained from the Dentist's Health Support Programme (formerly known as the Sick Dentist Scheme). Family support groups are a newly formed additional structure to the programme, developed because the spouse is recognised as an important aid to the resolution of the dentist's problems. The General Dental Council in the UK has procedures to protect patients while offering appropriate medical care (under the 1984 Dentists Act). Their responsibility is to ensure 'fitness to practise'. The Dentist Health and Support Group (tel. +44(0)207 487 3119) is a UK-based organisation that provides a service specifically for dentists. The Department of Health

UK Advisory Panel (tel. +44(0)207 7972 1529) provides guidelines on healthcare workers infected with blood-borne viruses.

Considering Change, Implementation and Coping

Problem-solving and goal-setting can be used to prevent and control occupational stress. By airing and discussing grievances, concerns and new strategies, members of the dental team can provide mutual support in times of stress. This has been called collective coping.

Stress does not occur in a vacuum, and it is important to avoid spiralling into repeated stressful experiences, which can lead to burn-out. The individual and preferably the team can:

- recognise the environmental demands
- assess and appraise the emotional consequences of these demands –for example, are they threatening, challenging, irrelevant or enhancing?
- adopt appropriate coping methods.

Planning for Retirement

As working life progresses the prospect of retirement edges closer. For some premature retirement is forced upon them due to illness. Dentists in their early forties are known to be four times more likely to retire prematurely than their colleagues in the medical profession. A national survey of 23,000 general medical practitioners in 2001 indicated that one in four intended to retire at the age of 55 to 57, and 80% reported they would retire at or before the age of 60. Reasons given for those who have taken early retirement are not easy to ascertain, as physical rather than mental illnesses are often preferred as explanations on medical reports. Burnout and mental illness feature in a sizeable proportion of dentists and can be the major factors for discontinuing work. Preventive approaches (for example, self-assessment, review of stressors and coping, seeking early support and mentoring), some of which have been mentioned previously, may reduce the numbers of dentists leaving their chosen profession due to illness.

In less extreme circumstances retirement can still be greeted with mixed emotions. New possibilities of a different and less hectic life-style beckon. For some, however, the hurdle of achieving the break from a lifetime's work appears onerous, if not insurmountable. Others may find the structure of the working week a vitally important part of their existence and prefer not to consider events post-retirement. A 'head-in-the-sand' approach can be viewed as avoidance and will have the propensity to increase uncertainty and anxiety about the future. As 73% of dentists in the UK and USA reach retirement age, the self-imposed neglect to consider this phase in the individual's life may have considerable negative consequences, such as reduced mood and financial insecurity. Active planning for retirement will prevent these anxieties and pressures. Apart from seeking financial advice well in advance of the retirement date, to include pension management and preparation of practice sale, for example, there are a number of other issues, some of them psychological, that require attention. These include:

- assessment of future goals – discuss with spouse, partner and dependents possible projects, activities (for example, sports, travelling, voluntary work or community ventures) and relate to current circumstances (financial, health and so on) and family responsibilities
- decide on whether to relocate or remain in the locality
- conduct a review of one's life from the perspective of 'self-actualisation', a term coined by the motivation expert, Maslow, referring to the extent that the individual feels they have achieved their major life goals.

Conclusions

This chapter has considered how the dentist may be prone to one of the most ubiquitous problems in modern-day living, that is occupational stress. Although dentists do not appear to be particularly unique in the levels reported, there is evidence that the nature of the job can be exacerbated by poor working conditions – for example, repetitive procedures, constant patient contact and a risk of errors unless a high level of concentration is maintained, and so on. The fact that many dentists are self-employed does not appear to be sufficiently protective. Hence, the value of self-assessment is advocated. Longer-term problems such as burnout are common if prolonged occupational stress is experienced. The prevention of these psychological problems and destructive methods of coping, such as drug or alcohol abuse, can be successfully applied with forethought and planning. The modern practitioner has many different resources to draw on, including local professional organisations (peer review and professional support groups, continuing professional development and electronic information sources).

The major tenet of this book has been to highlight the need to communicate effectively with patients, colleagues and staff. Good communication limits risks of patient/staff complaints and related problems. Effective communication enhances working relationships and ensures that, with parallel improvements in clinical skills, a balance can be achieved between technical excellence and the empathic and considered management of patients' oral health problems. Using the principles outlined in this book, dental health professionals can guarantee that their practice of dentistry remains a rewarding, satisfying and stress-free experience.

Further Reading

Websites for occupational stress
• Search engine with links to the topic of stress. www.healthfinder.gov
• A virtual library on stress. www.w3.org/vl/Stress/
• Comprehensive coverage of stress. www.cmhc.com/psyhelp/chap5/
• Holmes & Rahe stress test. www.prcn.org/next/stress.html

Websites for retirement planning
• Pre Retirement Association – an independent website for those considering early retirement – www.pra.uk.com/enter.html
• A further independent website – www.laterlife.com
• Recruits retired or semi-retired professionals for voluntary organisations www.volwork.org.uk

Cooper CL, Watts J, Kelly M. Job satisfaction, mental health, and job stressors among general dental practitioners in the UK. Br Dent J 1987;162:77-81.

Burke RJ, Greenglass ER. A longitudinal examination of the Cherniss model of psychological burnout. Soc Sci Med 1995;40:1357-1363.

Wilson RF, Coward PY, Capewell J et al. Perceived sources of occupational stress in general dental practitioners. British Dental Journal 1998;184;10:499-502.

Index

Quintessentials for General Dental Practitioners Series

in 50 volumes

Editor-in-Chief: Professor Nairn H F Wilson

General Dentistry, Editor: Nairn Wilson

Implantology in General Dental Practice	available
Cultural and Religious Issues in Clinical Practice	Spring 2006
Dilemmas of Dental Erosion	Spring 2006
Managing Orofacial Pain in Practice	Autumn 2006
Denatl Bleaching	Autumn 2006

Oral Surgery and Oral Medicine, Editor: John G Meechan

Practical Dental Local Anaesthesia	available
Practical Oral Medicine	available
Practical Conscious Sedation	available
Practical Surgical Dentistry	Spring 2006

Imaging, Editor: Keith Horner

Interpreting Dental Radiographs	available
Panoramic Radiology	Spring 2006
Twenty-first Century Dental Imaging	Autumn 2006

Periodontology, Editor: Iain L C Chapple

Understanding Periodontal Diseases: Assessment and Diagnostic Procedures in Practice	available
Decision-Making for the Periodontal Team	available
Successful Periodontal Therapy – A Non-Surgical Approach	available
Periodontal Management of Children, Adolescents and Young Adults	available
Periodontal Medicine: A Window on the Body	Spring 2006

Endodontics, Editor: John M Whitworth

Rational Root Canal Treatment in Practice	available
Managing Endodontic Failure in Practice	available
Preventing Pulpal Injury in Practice	Autumn 2006

Prosthodontics, Editor: P Finbarr Allen

Teeth for Life for Older Adults	available
Complete Dentures – from Planning to Problem Solving	available
Removable Partial Dentures	available
Fixed Prosthodontics in Dental Practice	available
Occlusion: A Theoretical and Team Approach	Autumn 2006

Operative Dentistry, Editor: Paul A Brunton

Decision-Making in Operative Dentistry	available
Aesthetic Dentistry	available
Communicating in Dental Practice	available
Indirect Restorations	Spring 2006
Choosing and Using Dental Materials	Autumn 2006

Paediatric Dentistry/Orthodontics, Editor: Marie Therese Hosey

Child Taming: How to Cope with Children in Dental Practice	available
Paediatric Cariology	available
Treatment Planning for the Developing Dentition	available
Managing Dental Trauma in Practice	available

General Dentistry and Practice Management, Editor: Raj Rattan

The Business of Dentistry	available
Risk Management	available
Quality Matters: From Clinical Care to Customer Service	Spring 2006
Practice Management for the Dental Team	Autumn 2006
Dental Practice Design	Autumn 2006
Handling Complaint in Dental Practice	Autumn 2006

Dental Team, Editor: Mabel Slater

Team Players in Dentistry	Spring 2006
Working with Dental Companies	Spring 2006
Getting it Right: Legal and Ethical Requirements for the Dental Team	Autumn 2006
Bridging the Communication Gap	Autumn 2006
Clinical Governance	Autumn 2006

Quintessence Publishing Co. Ltd., London